Celebrate Your Life

The optimistic guide to creating your own unique and truly personal funeral ceremony

Nicola Dela-Croix

Visit the author's website at www.nicoladelacroix.com

Cover by Stephanie Thannhauser
www.stephthannhauser.com

ISBN: 978-1-5272-3728-5

CONTENTS

1 WE ARE ALL UNIQUE

"And another regrettable thing about death is the ceasing of your own brand of magic…"
John Updike

A wonderful thing happened when you were born – you entered the world as a beautifully unique individual. There had never been anyone else like you on the planet before, and there never will be again. No-one else who walks this earth will ever look like you, sound like you, have the same special blend of characteristics, personality, qualities, tastes, experiences, relationships, achievements, challenges… the same life. You are a one off, never to be repeated. Isn't that incredible?

Your uniqueness was celebrated from the moment you arrived and it has set you apart at every single stage of your groundbreaking journey, from first steps and 'L' Plates, to finding your place in the big, wide world. And when this incredible life of yours draws to close, and your loved ones and friends gather together to give thanks for you and say farewell, that uniqueness should come alive in a final, meaningful reminder of the individual life you have led and the extraordinary person you have been.

Although you will probably have as much say in the timing of your departure as you did in your arrival, wouldn't it be nice to have some input in how you are remembered when the time comes? It was your life, after all. Those who shared in it will, of course, want to express their feelings, play their part, and reflect what you meant to them. But the real expert on you... is you. So if you want to ensure you have a funeral ceremony that is personal to you - one that reflects you honestly and accurately, celebrates your life and allows you to say farewell in your own style - then you need to give it some thought now. Plan ahead, express your wishes and share them while you are still here.

If the thought of planning your own funeral brings a feeling of gloom, doom and the tempting of fate, then stop right there. You have absolutely nothing to fear. Yes, we live in a society that doesn't like to think about lives ending or talk about funerals - we're still in denial about growing old, so coming to terms with the idea that one day we just won't be here any more is clearly a mind-blowing step too far! BUT it's a step we should all take, in spite of our fears. To help us get over this 'death is taboo' nonsense, we must embrace the idea of mortality and take control of how we are remembered. Then, not only will we get the truly personal funeral we deserve, we will also gain a whole new, positive perspective on life as we appreciate, more than ever, that our time is limited and precious.

We have to make the most of the years we have and appreciate our unique value in the world while we are still part of it. So the more we shy away from talking about death and the prospect of our own funeral, the more we are denying ourselves the chance to live the full, all-embracing, wide-screen, technicolour life that only exists when you know it's not forever.

A unique life needs a unique send off. We owe it to ourselves, to our family and friends to make that happen. But you will need help, and that's where this book comes in. As a Funeral Celebrant, I've spent the last decade creating hundreds of unique funeral ceremonies for unique people – people of all ages, backgrounds and beliefs. Many of these people were unknown to me, while others I'd met in the final stages of terminal illness. It's a big, beautiful list of over 1,000 individuals that I've had the pleasure of talking about - celebrating their lives and helping loved-ones say goodbye. It's a huge privilege I don't take lightly.

And out of all those ceremonies, the ones that I remember most have been the ones with the personal touches that, on the day, have so much meaning. The rescue dog volunteer with a guard of honour made up of greyhounds, who gently and quietly stood to attention as her coffin arrived. The knitting Nanna whose floral tribute consisted of woollen flowers hand-made by her daughters and granddaughters. The teenager whose coffin was decorated with photographs, multi-coloured messages and the glitter handprints of her friends. I've handed out lily bulbs on behalf of a keen gardener, golf balls for a sportsman, watched friends waltz around the crematorium chapel as they remembered their dancing school teacher. Then there are the special locations – trees planted in gardens, glasses raised in favourite pubs, tributes paid, and tea and cake shared, in village halls. And all the photographic slideshows I've watched, recorded messages listened to and last letters read.

Some of those wishes were carried out at the deceased's request, others were gestures from family and friends – their last opportunity to do something for this special person they knew and loved. And that's the combination which seems to work best and prove to be so memorable – when we are remembering a life in the way that person wished, AND the people they have left behind are able to contribute and show their love in a way that brings them comfort.

And as a Celebrant I'm there to bring everything together, to capture the essence of this special person and help their loved-ones express what they can't always put into words. To leave them knowing their mum, dad, daughter, brother, friend had 'a good send-off' - their journey of life rounded off with a fitting farewell they themselves would have approved of, and everyone there enjoyed. Yes, you can 'enjoy' a funeral. People often lean in secretively and say to me after a ceremony "I know I shouldn't say this but I really enjoyed that". And why shouldn't they? If I've done my job properly on the day then we will have remembered someone with the same love and happiness they themselves knew in life. There are sadder moments, of course, as we acknowledge their loss in a dignified and respectful way, but with that loss comes an appreciation of all that was gained when they were part of our world, however long or short that stay was.

So now, I'm combining all my skills and experience to show you exactly how to create a truly personal and unique life celebration for yourself - taking away the fear, busting the myths and clearing the confusion that can be associated with funeral ceremonies. And, if you follow this process, by the end you will not only have a tailor-made funeral ceremony, but also a new-found appreciation for life itself, for the person you are, the value you hold in the world and in the lives of others. Can we have an outcome of 'feel good' and 'funeral ceremony' in the same book? Absolutely!

2 THERE IS NOTHING TO FEAR

"Nothing in life is to be feared. It is only to be understood. Now is the time to understand more, so that we may fear less"
Marie Curie

A huge benefit of thinking about and planning funeral ceremonies in advance is that you are not only prepared and well-informed, but your loved-ones will also be armed with the information they will need when the time comes. And they will be extremely grateful for that. Because there is a 'system' in place that most of us experience and become part of when a loved-one dies, from registering the death to making arrangements with a firm of funeral directors. It's really important that we feel in control of this process that can seem as overwhelming as it is unfamiliar - grief knocks us sideways, so having to think, plan, and make decisions at such a time will take gargantuan effort. And all that thinking, planning and decision-making won't come at a pace that is gentle. There is approximately a fortnight, on average, from death to funeral. And if your family has absolutely no idea what your wishes were, then they will also feel the weight of wondering if the choices they make for you are the right ones.

I trained as a funeral arranger and worked for a local funeral director before becoming a Celebrant. So I know exactly what it's like to sit with a newly-bereaved family who don't even know if their mum, dad, husband, daughter wanted to be buried or cremated, and how distressing that is for them. It's the most basic of questions and most people, when asked, usually feel quite strongly one way or the other. But if the 'burial or cremation' question was never asked during this person's lifetime, or the wish never expressed, how will they know? And alongside that decision, they will be asked about where they want the funeral to be, who will lead it, do they need cars, what coffin would they like, and how about flowers, orders of service, donations, refreshments afterwards…

So many things to think about… and that's just the start. After that initial meeting with a funeral arranger, they will then have a meeting with the person who is leading the ceremony. Someone like me. And I will be asking them all about you - where you were born, how you got on at school, your working life, interests, what you were passionate about, proudest moments, who were the special people in your life, how can we describe your character and personality, what music you liked, did you have any favourite poems or books, how would you like to be remembered…

Do you really want to leave all that to your loved-ones without any input, information or help from you in advance? And do you want to be in the same position when you have to plan a funeral for a member of your own family? I do my best not to make people feel like they are being bombarded with questions or pressured to make decisions - in fact, the experience of talking about someone you have loved and lost can be extremely comforting and very often there is as much laughter as tears when we get together. BUT it is still a huge amount of information to share and process, and all at time when even switching the kettle on is an effort.

The more you, and your family, know in advance, the easier this highly emotional experience will be. And that's where I come in. My area of expertise is meaningful, personal funeral ceremonies - life celebrations. So before I take away that fear of the unknown and show you how to create one that is right for you, let me tell you what I think are the essential elements of a good funeral ceremony. These elements are based on my experiences of creating and leading hundreds of funeral ceremonies, the reactions I see and hear from people gathered on the day, and the feedback I get from families afterwards.

A MEANINGFUL CEREMONY...

1. Captures the essence of the person

The most important and fulfilling challenge of my work as a Celebrant is to accurately and honestly capture the life, personality and uniqueness of each person. When a family invite me into their home, during the saddest time of their life, and share with me their stories and memories of this special person they knew and loved, I have to do them justice. In fact, I make it my mission to ensure those stories and experiences, all those quirks and characteristics are captured and shared on the day in a meaningful, accurate way. And those little quirks are important because recalling them creates the moments during a ceremony when I can see people nod their head and smile, or laugh. It's the little details about a person that bring them to life - how they liked milky tea, not answering the phone when Emmerdale is on, always buying yellow motorbikes... So when someone says to me after a ceremony "how long had you known Dave?" or "that was Alice to a T" or "Mum would have loved it" then I know I've got it right.

2. Has the input of the deceased and their loved-ones

The most memorable and meaningful funeral ceremonies are the ones where we are honouring someone's life in the way they wished to be remembered AND the people they have left behind are able to contribute in a way that brings them comfort. Being able to say to everyone "we've come together to celebrate Jill's life, as that was her wish for today" sets a lovely tone from the very beginning of the ceremony, making everyone feel they are playing a part that day in remembering Jill in the way she wanted - the last thing they can do for her. And alongside fulfilling Jill's wish is the opportunity for her family and friends to express their own feelings of love and gratitude for having known her and shared in her life, either through tributes shared, flowers chosen and music selected.

3. Reflects the feelings of those who knew and loved them

There are times during a ceremony, when the feelings of love and affection for the person who has died are so strong, so palpable, I think the roof is going to lift off or the windows explode. When happy memories are being shared and everyone is laughing out loud, or music is being listened to and tears silently run, that's when I look at the coffin and I think to myself, I really hope this person knew just how much they meant to all these people - how much their life mattered and how special they were. And you don't have to have a room full of people to get that same sense of appreciation. I've done ceremonies where there have been two or three people present, sometimes care home staff who looked after someone who had no family or had outlived them. And their memories of looking after this person and how they made them laugh, or their admiration as they remember the dignity they showed throughout their illness, can be just as moving. So it's the sharing of those memories - as well as expressing feelings - that are essential in order to reflect the impact someone has had in the lives of others.

4. Focuses on the beliefs and wishes of the deceased and their family

Funerals cannot always be neatly divided into religious or non-religious. Yes, if you have lived your life with a strong faith, then a fully religious funeral ceremony is fitting for you. Alternatively, if you had no faith at all, then a non-religious ceremony is more appropriate. But there are lots of people who fall somewhere in the middle - they weren't church-goers but would appreciate a prayer, they loved singing along to Songs of Praise and carols at Christmas, or had a hymn at their wedding which holds special meaning and memories. Some people refer to themselves as spiritual rather than religious, so a reading or quote that fits those spiritual beliefs is fitting on the day. The first question I ask when discussing what type of funeral is fitting for someone is not - were they religious or not? I start by asking… who were they? What sort of person, how did they live their life, what was important to them? And from those questions, we can piece together a picture of a unique person, and what their individual beliefs and wishes were, then build a unique ceremony around them.

5. Is in the right venue

Depending on the style of ceremony you want, and whether you are being buried or cremated, venues currently include churches, crematorium chapels, burial ground chapels or graveside services. I've also led ceremonies in village halls, hotel and pub function rooms, community centres and private gardens. For some people, the venue for the ceremony itself is hugely significant and that takes priority, while for others it's more about practicality for the ceremony and the refreshments afterwards are in a more personal place. Sometimes the content of the ceremony is restricted if, for example, there are no audiovisual facilities at a village hall, or the crematorium has a short time slot, but my job is to ensure that, wherever the ceremony takes place, it's as special as it can be.

6. Brings people together

Sounds pretty obvious but that sense of togetherness - being part of that uniquely special circle of family, friends, colleagues, classmates who all have one person is common - is a beautiful thing. At some point during the journey of that person's life, their path crossed with others, relationships were formed, friendships shared and memories made. So being together to share in honouring this person's life, and the part you played in it, is an essential aspect of what makes a meaningful ceremony. And, of course, being there to support and comfort each other.

7. Is as original and unique as the person themselves

I pride myself on the fact that I have never done the same ceremony twice. Sometimes there are themes, phrases, or quotes, that are ideally suited for particular circumstances, for example remembering a young person who has died suddenly. And there can be a particular order in which I do things - and this is based on me coming up with an 'order of service' that I think will provide the most meaning and comfort to people on the day. But even with similar circumstances and running orders, every ceremony I create begins with a blank sheet and that's how it should be.

8. Includes personal touches

There are so many ways to include personal touches to a funeral ceremony. I mentioned some of them in the previous chapter - the knitted flowers, greyhound guard of honour and decorated coffin. You can design your own order of service sheets or ask everyone to wear your favourite colour. I was even asked to start a ceremony a few minutes late because this particular lady never arrived anywhere on time. When I explained why the ceremony was late, it brought recognition and laughter. A lovely way to begin proceedings.

9. Makes the most of audio-visual opportunities

The world of funerals is a slow one, in terms of technological advances. But this is largely due to many of the venues being quite old and, possibly, an outdated concern that being too modern or making too many changes too quickly will upset traditionalists and perhaps seem disrespectful. But as far as I'm concerned, there are ways of making ceremonies both respectful and be a true representation of people's lives and personal wishes. We must move with the times and reflect the needs of modern families and individuals. Happily these days most crematoriums have the facility to download music, show photographic montages or videos on a large TV screen, provide live webcasts and record ceremonies for people who cannot attend. Done well, and at the right point in the ceremony, these audio-visual additions can be both uplifting and moving in equal measure, a multi-sensory experience taking ceremonies to a new, much more meaningful level.

10. Tells you something about the person you didn't already know

We all mean different things to different people. And all those unique relationships and strands of a person's life should be reflected in some way on the day. The beauty of that is two-fold. Firstly, everyone will feel included in some way as their special connection to this person is acknowledged. Secondly, people will find out something about their loved one or friend they didn't know. Those lovely stories and memories are also shared in the cards of condolence or Facebook messages left in the days before and after the ceremony. I often ask families during a visit to their home if they would mind sharing some of the messages in their sympathy cards which are displayed around the room. They are always happy to do so, grateful for the opportunity to share what their loved-one meant to others. And it gives me a chance to see that person from a perspective outside their family. I remember a lovely lady who was crying with laughter at some of the messages sent by her husband's work colleagues, telling tales of his pranks and the laughs they had in the factory where he worked. We shared some of them on the day. Wonderful stuff...

11. Acknowledges grief and the sense of loss

Capturing the essence of a person, and reflecting what they meant to others, is one challenge. I also have to strike a very delicate balance between expressing everyone's sense of loss with a sense of gratitude for the fact that they were fortunate to have had this person in their life, for however long. That is something they must take comfort in and give thanks for. Because grief goes hand in hand with love - you can't have one without the other. So it's important to include all those feelings in a way that is manageable for people. So they know we appreciate the pain that comes from having to say goodbye to someone you love, but also provide comfort with reminders of shared love, happy days, and memories that will outlive their goodbyes.

12. Includes smiles and laughter

No matter how tragic the circumstances, there should be moments in every ceremony where people are able to smile and laugh. That's in no way disrespectful because we are remembering someone's life – a life which experienced its share of happiness and humour, its own little quirks or funny sayings. Even lives that were over before they had a chance to begin. I've done ceremonies for babies, including stillborn babies. And alongside the parent's pain of those dashed hopes were opportunities to express gratitude for the moments when their little one still made their presence felt. Such as the mummy smiling at the memory of carrying her little 'Tigger' who wouldn't keep still, and who seemed to be waving in all her scan photographs. There was a ripple of gentle laughter on the day when I shared those memories. Heart-breaking and heart-warming in equal measure. That mummy stayed in touch with me, and sent me a picture of her new baby when she arrived 18 months later.

13. Has a sense of 'gravitas'

I've talked about the need for ceremonies to include a meaningful mix of expressing loss and celebrating life. We also need to keep a sense of occasion - to have moments which bring gravitas, a dignified air to proceedings. These include asking people to stand when the coffin enters the chapel and again during the committal. For me to bow at the coffin when it arrives at the venue and again before I leave the room. It keeps things respectful - a reminder that this person who walked the earth is now leaving it. Respect and attention is required. And everyone deserves a dignified farewell.

14. Has someone to lead proceedings

You're probably thinking "well she would say that, wouldn't she!" but this isn't me making myself indispensable. Whatever type of ceremony you have, and wherever you have it, you need someone on the day who is going to co-ordinate the ceremony, set the right tone, welcome everyone, cue the music, deliver the right words at the right time, express what others find hard to say, introduce any other speakers and bring everything together. Preferably someone who is not emotionally attached to the deceased, can speak well and strike that balance between mourning a loss and celebrating a life. Someone who can deal with the unexpected, and keep to time. And, of course, someone the family have already met and are comfortable with.

15. Is memorable…

A good funeral ceremony will stay in people's minds for a very long time. Unfortunately, the same can be said for a bad ceremony. The unexpected can happen - from small technical hitches where I've cued the music only to be met with silence, to the more dramatic as one poor man had a heart attack in front of me as he was reading a tribute to his sister (he was taken to hospital and recovered, thankfully). Some things are avoidable, others aren't. But the more you put into the planning and organisation of a ceremony, the more chances you have of it running smoothly and being memorable... for all the right reasons.

16. Is rounded off with food and drink

Whether it's tea and cake, or beer and a buffet, gathering together for refreshments after the ceremony is the ideal opportunity for people to continue sharing their memories in a more relaxed environment, and to catch up with family and friends they perhaps haven't seen for years, or even met before. It's a chance for everyone to keep that celebration of life going beyond the confines of a church or chapel, in a space often chosen for personal reasons – the family home, a favourite watering hole, a team sports club. Sometimes the refreshments are seen as more important than the ceremony - on more than one occasion I've been told the deceased specifically asked that the funeral be kept as short as possible so everyone can get to the pub afterwards! And there is nothing more heart-warming than seeing groups of people gathered together, starting sentences with "Do you remember the time…" and heads thrown back in laughter.

17. Makes you appreciate life

A good funeral ceremony not only makes you appreciate the life of someone you have known and loved, but it makes you appreciate your own life too. And the lives of the people close to you. I don't know about you, but every time I come out of a funeral I take a deep breath, look at the trees and the sky, absorb all the wonderful signs of life and think 'I'm so glad I'm still here'. My role as a Celebrant isn't to preach to people, but I do make an effort, in every ceremony, to sensitively communicate the fact that life is precious, people are precious, and none of us know how long we have to embrace both. So when we come together to celebrate a life, we are giving thanks for our lives, as well as the lives of others.

****

That's quite a list isn't it? But don't be overwhelmed! The whole point of this book is to gently guide you through this process, bringing together your own thoughts and wishes which will combine to create a ceremony with all these essential elements. And while the focus is on helping you put together your own celebration of life, you can, of course, use the information to create a ceremony for loved-ones and friends.

You may be thinking, what if I don't want a funeral ceremony? Well, that's absolutely fine. As far as the official, legal requirement goes your death has to be registered and your body has to be disposed of, but aside from that, you are not required to have a funeral at all if you don't want one. David Bowie didn't want a funeral. His wishes were for a private cremation shortly after his death and his ashes scattered in Bali in line with Buddhist rituals - no fuss, no funeral. And that's exactly what happened, his wishes were fulfilled. But it didn't stop his family from mourning his loss or remembering him in their own private way. And it certainly didn't stop his musical contemporaries and worldwide fans from paying their own tributes. I'm a fan too and had my own moments of listening to his music, and talking about him with friends, in the days after his death. And that's the beauty of Bowie's legacy – we can still hear him and watch him, even though he's no longer a physical part of the world.

Whether your legacy is great or small, whether you have done something extraordinary or you have led a simple, quiet life and just want a simple, quiet exit to go with it, as long as your wishes are expressed and then carried out, that's all that matters. So make sure you let your family know. They may not feel comfortable, initially, of letting you go without a ceremony – it may feel too impersonal, too clinical, and what about their opportunity to gather together and see you on your way with love? Well, they can still gather together at another time or place, still share memories, still express what you've meant to them and raise a glass to you. In fact, that's what most of us continue to do in the days, months and years after someone we love has died. We are continually remembering. You don't have to be a Rock Star to live on in the hearts and minds of others.

3 REMEMBER ME: HOW TO CREATE YOUR OWN LIFE CELEBRATION

So how would you like to be remembered? And how can you make your farewell ceremony as meaningful to you as it will be for your family and friends? Using my knowledge and experience as a Funeral Celebrant, I've created a two-part process which encourages you to think about these questions and helps you find some answers. The result is your own collection of farewell wishes for a truly personal celebration of life. These wishes can then be shared with your loved ones in person, or simply placed with important documents so they can be found when needed. And, of course, you can change or add to your wishes at any time, keeping them as relevant and up to date as possible.

There are two parts to Remember Me because we can't leap in to creating a life celebration without first appreciating the life behind the ceremony. So Part One - 'Your Life' - is all about you - who you are, what you've done, who with, the memories you've made… And in Part Two - 'Your Ceremony' - we combine all that information and start piecing together the ceremony itself. Both parts go into detail, with lots of questions, prompts, information and ideas. But again, do not be overwhelmed! You can answer and decide on as much, or as little, as you like, whenever you like. And, as I'm hoping you will have plenty of years still ahead of you, your life will change in time, and your wishes may change with it, so it's something you can come back to whenever you feel like it.

This is one of the most positive things you can do for yourself and your loved ones. You will know you are being remembered in a fitting way that means something to you, and your family will take comfort in being able to fulfill your wishes. And, taking time out to focus on the end of your life will indeed give a wonderful, new, uplifting perspective on who you are, the life you have lived and the years you still have to come. So be courageous and make those all-important decisions while you can.

****

Before we begin, here are some thoughts on how you may wish to capture all of this valuable information...

Capturing your life story and wishes
When I learnt to type at school in the 80's, it was the era of the electronic typewriter, using a carbon sheet between two pieces of paper so you could send a letter and keep one copy for yourself. Fast forward to the 90's, when I became a journalist, and I was introduced to the first Apple Mac computer. Not only could you could correct as you went along but you could print as many copies as you like… mind blowing! Well it was at the time...

Yes, technology has come a long way since the 80's and it continues to progress at high speed. So while using your desktop computer, laptop or some other digital device to type up your life story and express your wishes, you'll no doubt also have access to all sorts of software that will allow you to create a multi-media, all-singing, all-dancing, creation with pictures, music, video, links etc. added in to the mix. There's no point even naming any of these applications because a) I'm no techie and b) it will be out of date by the time you read this. But if you have the time, inclination and the know-how, the world is your lobster!

Alternatively…
You may wish to keep things simple and opt for a notebook and pen. And who can blame you? In this age of keyboards and touch screens there is something intensely satisfying about writing by hand. Getting your thoughts down can feel cathartic, nostalgic even. It's also very personal, reflecting another aspect

of your individuality as your handwriting fills the page. And if that notebook should be left for your loved ones, think how much more of a treasure it will be for them to see words in your own hand, rather than a cold computerised typeface.

Get Creative

Do you remember having a scrapbook as a kid? Sticking in all sorts of things and then the joy of flicking through the pages once they were filled? Well, you can create your own 'memory book' of your life story. This could be a lovely collection of words, images, and also memorabilia, such as travel tickets or music festival programmes, whatever you like. You then get to enjoy it in the years to come and leave it for others to enjoy when your story draws to a close.

Sound and Vision

I mentioned how unique our handwriting is, and how it reflects our individuality. The same can be said of our voices and, most definitely, our faces. So a life story and farewell wishes captured in an audio or video recording gives your story a whole new dimension. Hearing the voice of someone dearly departed, or seeing their face in front of you once again, is a gift technology has made possible for everyone, even with just the swipe of a smartphone. It can certainly play a meaningful part on the day as we celebrate your life. How .great to be able to use technology in such a life-affirming, positive way.

So if you're ready, let's begin!

4 REMEMBER ME
PART ONE: YOUR LIFE

Celebration of 'Life'... the clue is in the title. If you want a personal funeral ceremony, we have to get personal. Over six different stages you'll have the opportunity to capture the story of your life in words, images and music, recognise your achievements, celebrate your uniqueness, appreciate your precious place in the world and in the lives of others. Those are big subjects and you are in control of how much you wish to reflect on and what you want share with others.

Having the opportunity to think about all those aspects of your life can be an uplifting and meaningful journey in itself, giving you a sharper focus on where your life has taken you and where you'd like it to go next. And not only does the information you gather here form the basis of Part Two, as we put together your life celebration ceremony, it can also be presented as a memento to your loved-ones, who would, I'm sure, appreciate your own perspective on 'you' - the person they have known and loved.

The six stages we'll go through are...

ONE: YOUR LIFE STORY
We all have our own story to tell, and we begin by drawing an outline of your unique life so far – where you've come from, where you are now and all the events and experiences in-between. Plus inspiration from the life stories of others.

TWO: YOUR RELATIONSHIPS
You've not been alone in your story and Stage Two is all about the people who have shared in the journey of your life, lived alongside you, and how meaningful they have been. Plus the significance of ancestors and the people keeping our memory alive in the future.

THREE: MEMORABLE MOMENTS
We look at the good, the proud, the challenging, and the eventful moments in your life that have been memorable to you. We reflect on why they mattered, what their impact has been and what you've learnt from them..

FOUR: MUSIC AND MEMENTOS
What music has featured in the soundtrack to your life? What photographs have best captured you and your story? What prized possessions could you never be parted from? We'll look at these all-important collections in Section Four and how they fit into the story of your life.

FIVE: THE UNIQUE YOU
You are a one-off, never-to-be-repeated individual. And that incredible fact is something to celebrate. So here we look at what sets you apart, from how you look and behave, to your personality, qualities and values. We also get an outside perspective and look at which unique individuals have inspired you.

SIX: ONWARD JOURNEYS
In our final part we highlight what this journey through your life story has uncovered, what you've learnt from it and how you might like to share that wisdom. We look ahead to the years to come and focus on what you'd like to do more of, and end with some positive thoughts before moving on to Part Two - 'Your Ceremony'.

SECTION ONE
Your Life Story

"In the end we'll all become stories"
Margaret Atwood

Life Stories… they are everywhere, happening around us every second of every day. We live our own life story, we share it with the life stories of those we know – our family, friends, colleagues and neighbours – and we watch life stories happening to people we don't know – strangers on trains, couples in cafes, families on holiday. We follow life stories in television dramas, on the news and in social media. We read about life stories in books – lives imagined and created, lives past and present. We admire other lives, find inspiration and hope in them…

Your story is woven into this rich tapestry of life. It interconnects in all sorts of wonderful, colourful ways. It is experienced, shared, watched, and admired. It reaches out and touches the lives of others. It makes its unique mark. And it holds meaning in more ways than you'll ever know. There is certainly no such thing as an 'ordinary' life. I've had the privilege of writing and sharing hundreds of life stories through my work as a Celebrant. And while some have appeared, on paper, to be more eventful than others, there isn't one life story that hasn't made a positive impression on me in one way or another.

In this first section, we're going to look at your own life story starting with the main events of your life, ie. where you were born, where you lived and went to school, what work you've done, what interests you've had… Basically drawing an outline of your life so far, together with relevant anecdotes and memories. This will form the basis of your story which we will refer back to in future stages of this creative process, as we elaborate and fill in more of the colours, looking at relationships, memorable moments, your personal, musical soundtrack, and, of course, when we go on to create your ceremony.

Questions to ask

For the past however many years, you have been living your life. And that life will have consisted of some, or all, of the following – being born, growing up, going to school, making friends, working, falling in love, raising a family, travelling, reading, listening, watching, doing... This life has been unique to you, no-one else. It's all yours. So what do you remember about it? What have been the main events and experiences? It's entirely up to you how detailed you want to be and whether you want to approach things chronologically or by subject, ie. Childhood, Working Life, Family, etc.

Here are some questions to help you along...

Early Life and Education

- Where and when were you born?
- What are your parents' names?
- Do you have brothers and sisters?
- Where did you grow up?
- What do you remember most about your childhood?
- Who were your friends?
- Did you have family holidays?
- What schools did you go to?
- What subjects did you enjoy/excel in?
- Did you go on to further education? College or University?
- What qualifications did you gain?
- Were there any formative experiences that influenced your choice of career?

Relationships

- What have been your most significant relationships – both past and present – ie. with parents, siblings, spouses, partners, children, grandchildren, friends?
- Have you been married? Do you have a partner?
- Do you have children? Grandchildren?
- Who are your friends?
- Have you had pets?
- Who are you closest to?

Working Life

- When did you start working?
- Did you have paper rounds or Saturday jobs to earn pocket money?
- What was your first full-time job?
- Where has your working life taken you since then?
- Who have you worked with in terms of both organisations and people?
- Have you ever been self-employed?
- Have you ever done voluntary work?
- What work qualifications, skills and experience have you gained along the way?
- Which colleagues or managers stand out in your memory?

Interests

- Do you have any particular interests or hobbies? If so, what are they?
- Have you travelled? If so, where? Which trips stand out, and why?
- Any strong likes or dislikes of yours?
- Do you have any particular talents or skills?

Anecdotes and Stories

Alongside the relevant dates, names and places, it's a good idea to include any specific memories, anecdotes and stories as you go along. Because it's those memories – calling to mind what you experienced and how you felt – that hold more meaning to you. They provide the colour within the outline of your life and make your story unique and interesting. And, of course, these memories and stories can be shared as part of your life celebration, and they will live on after you, in the hearts and minds of loved ones who shared in those moments.

Not all your stories will be richly detailed or even particularly eventful. Sometimes it's the simplest things about your life that become significant, as you can see from the following examples. These are short extracts from real-life stories I've shared during funeral ceremonies. I have, however, changed the names…

When Kate and Dave started dating in May 1976 they missed out on seeing the then relatively unknown Sex Pistols. Given the choice of two pubs, they opted for the one that didn't have such a racket going on inside.

Sarah excelled at long jump – she was so good, in fact, that she jumped the full length of the long jump pit at school and it had to be closed for Health & Safety reasons until she left.

Cycling to work, Bill knocked out his pipe tobacco on the cycle frame, and set his socks on fire.

Maureen worked as an usherette at the cinema – complete with torch and ice cream tray. She always told the story of how she saw the film Paint Your Wagon about 70 times but always missed the same bit because she had to fetch the ice creams.

Ron absolutely loved his garden – he was even known to come home from work at night and rig up a torch on the washing line so he could tend his veg in the dark.

THE LIVES OF OTHERS - 5 LIVES IN BOOKS

We engage in life stories in all sorts of ways, from the music we listen to and films we watch, to books we read and places we visit. Some of those life stories stay with us, striking a chord and making an impact in their own meaningful way. From my first copy of 'Miffy Goes Flying', books have been a joy to me and I cannot imagine life without them. Everyone has their own preferences, but here are five autobiographies that have a special place in my heart and my book case...

Little House in the Big Woods by Laura Ingalls Wilder
The first (and my favourite) of the Little House on the Prairie series about an American pioneering family in the late 19th century seen through the eyes of Laura. I still have the original set of books from my childhood and they are so charming and have such a vivid sense of history I recently re-read them all again.

Greetings from Bury Park by Sarfraz Manzoor
Sarfraz came to Britain from Pakistan as a small child and these are his memories of growing up in Bury Park, Luton. It's both moving and funny, as he talks about his parents, his dreams for the future and his passion for the music of Bruce Springsteen. I grew up about 15 miles from Sarfraz and my father also came to England from India – so it struck an emotive chord with me. This book was also released as a film, re-named Blinded By The Light, in 2019.

A Handful of Earth by Barney Bardsley
Barney is a woman whose husband was diagnosed with cancer when he was 36. After he died, and with their very young daughter to support, Barney finds solace in her allotment. And gradually, plant by plant, month by month, and season by season her life begins to restore itself. This book left me feeling uplifted, grateful and with a deep desire to get out into the garden.

Swan River by David Reynolds

This is a beautiful, beautiful book about three generations – a son (the author, David Reynolds), father and grandfather – stretching back more than a century. I was so caught up in this family and the feelings between them, that I was torn between gorging myself on one chapter after another, and pacing myself because I didn't want it to end. Everything a good book should be.

Star Gazing by Peter Hill

Peter was a Dundee College of Art student in the 1970's when he answered a newspaper advert seeking lighthouse keepers. Within a month he was living with three men he didn't know in a lighthouse on a remote island off the West Coast of Scotland. This is a fantastic memoir of his time there, and on other lighthouses, the eclectic people he met, and his feelings for a simpler way of life, now gone. I adored this book and reading it while I was on holiday on the Scottish West Coast added to its charm.

SECTION TWO
Your Relationships

"I am a part of all that I have met"
Alfred, Lord Tennyson

Every single person on the planet has a life inextricably intertwined with others. Even if you've spent your entire life as a hermit in the remotest of caves, shut off from society and civilisation, someone still gave birth to you. From mums and dads, brothers and sisters, grandparents, aunties, uncles, cousins, husbands, wives, partners, sons, daughters, to friends, teachers, colleagues, neighbours... we experience a wide and wonderful range of relationships. And that's just the people we know!

More human beings than we could possibly imagine have been aware of our existence. What about all the people we don't count as family, friends or acquaintances who have somehow played a part in our lives, like doctors and driving instructors? And how about all those brief encounters we experience every day – a morning wave to a fellow dog walker, a chat about the weather with a fellow bus passenger?

All these relationships have had an impact on our lives – some in a far more meaningful way than others. And as the years have gone by, the way we conduct these relationships, communicate and interact with people has changed dramatically, especially in the last decade or two. That's bad news if you liked receiving handwritten letters, but good news if you have loved ones in Australia who Skype you once a week…

So now we're going to look at the people who have shared in your life. Using the life story you put together in Section One, you can identify who has shared in your journey so far. You won't, of course, remember everyone – some names and faces will frustratingly elude you while others take you by surprise as they pop into your mind. You'll also think about which of your relationships have been the most significant and meaningful, and who you are grateful to have shared the planet with. And we'll look at ancestors who link us to the past and the people who will keep our memory alive in the future.

Who have you shared your life with?

That's quite a big question, so let's break it down a bit. There are two ways of approaching this, just as we did with your life story – in date order or subject matter. At this point we're looking at the people you know, who you've shared a relationship with, so that will include family, friends, neighbours, teachers, colleagues, etc. It doesn't matter how many names you get down, or who you do and don't remember. You might just want to focus on your immediate family. There's no right or wrong way of doing this. Remember – you can do as much or as little of each section as you like, it's entirely up to you - it's your life, your story. And it's a story which continues – new people will come into your life and others will leave – so it's all a moveable feast.

Chronological
Using dates and/or ages, make a note of the people who were part of your life at that time. Use your life story to remind yourself where you were living and what you were doing.

Subject Matter
You might prefer to think in terms of groups of people. Such as...

Family – immediate and extended, the family you grew up with – parents, siblings, grandparents, aunties, uncles, cousins...Significant others – husbands, wives, partners, girlfriends, boyfriends.

Offspring – your children, grandchildren, great-grandchildren
Friends – who you grew up with, studied with, worked with, shared interests, holidays and nights out.
Neighbours – from chatting over the fence to a friend in need
Teachers – the good, the bad and the inspirational
Colleagues – team work, office banter, Christmas parties.
Pets - the furry, four-legged companions you'll never forget.

Some of these people will still be part of your life, others will be out of touch but still out there in the world somewhere, and some will have reached the end of their story. The point is to recognise and appreciate how your life has been intertwined with the lives of others, and those who have made the most impact…

"Be careful who you make memories with. Those things can last a lifetime"

Family Stories

"Family means no-one gets left behind or forgotten."
David Ogden Stiers

When you work as a Funeral Celebrant, it's abundantly clear how important family is to people. It's rare to have a ceremony without mention of the special part someone played in the lives of their loved ones – a much-loved dad, a loyal and loving wife, a proud mum, a thoughtful son… Sometimes, when I visit families, the desire to focus on these roles is so strong, it's difficult to shift the conversation onto other areas of life, such as work, interests or character and qualities. But it's understandable – the focus on family gives everyone left behind a sense of having shared a meaningful connection with this person. A relationship that was both part of the wider family, and uniquely personal to the two of them.

Needless to say not all families are close and not everyone shares the same level of grief – funerals, like weddings, can reveal cracks in a family and, sometimes, widen those divisions. I do have to tread very carefully at times. But, every week, I will lead at least one ceremony that really encapsulates all that's joyful and positive about being part of a tribe. Where the love and appreciation for this deeply missed person, their little quirks and well-known ways, their special place within the family, is recognised and celebrated, sometimes in the simplest of ways, like this…

Ethel didn't become a great-nan until later in life. And when identical twins Lauren and Louis paid her a visit at the Care Home, Ethel said "Look! Buy one get one free!"

Stan's parents were not wealthy people, but sometimes they managed a holiday to the coast. On one occasion his mum and dad boarded the coach and, on arriving at their destination, realised they had left him and his younger brother at the bus stop in Dorking!

Sylvia was fiercely intelligent, proudly independent and utterly unorthodox. Her daughters cringed at this when they were younger – as their mother would arrive at the school gates with a Victorian fur stole thrown nonchalantly around her shoulders, compared to their friend's mothers who were more conservatively dressed in twin-sets and pearls. But as they grew older they were more grateful for Sylvia's eccentricity – they loved the fact that their mum was a little different.

As big brother, it was Stu's job to look after his young sister Sarah. She recalls he would take her swimming or to buy sweets, always in the knowledge that she was 'cramping his style'. He even took her along to see this favourite rock band, Deep Purple, for her 14th birthday.

On Rachel's Wedding Day, everyone else left for the church and she was alone with her Dad. He told her how beautiful she looked then realised how scared and nervous she was. So he poured her a tot of neat Southern Comfort to try to calm her down. It didn't work, but certainly gave her cheeks a bit of colour.

The evening Reg's new grandson came home, Reg proudly arrived, camera in hand. It had taken several hours to settle little Noah, so his parents said to Reg "Whatever you do dad, do not use the flash". "Oh it's alright" says Reg, "one won't hurt". It was 4am before Noah settled again…

Who made a difference?

"At times our own light goes out and is rekindled by a spark from another person. Each of us has cause to think with deep gratitude of those who have lighted the flame within us."
Albert Schweitzer

Relationships are complex and colourful. Some bring joy and happiness, while others cause pain and heartache. Some take us off in new, adventurous directions, others provide stability and familiarity. Some are for life, others just a short chapter in the story – even the briefest of moments. But whatever the diversities, all these relationships have the ability to teach us something about life and about ourselves. That does, of course, make the question 'who made a difference' an easy one to answer because everyone, in their own way added something, even if it was a lesson in what not to do.

So take a moment to look through your list of names. In addition to your immediate family and the people who are closest to you, do any others stand out as being particularly meaningful? Was there a teacher who encouraged you towards your chosen career path? A grandparent whose values and wisdom inspired you? A friend who stepped in when your spouse walked out? A bad boss who forced that job change which turned out to be the best move you ever made? Highlight these names, make a note of the difference they made to you and your life.

Close encounters with the unknown

This is not about UFO's or other unexplained phenomena. I'm referring to strangers you crossed paths with at some stage in the journey of your life, individuals who did something or said something which meant a great deal at the time. It could be as significant as someone rushing to your rescue when you had an accident, or as simple as someone sharing their loose change at a parking meter. Big or small acts of kindness showing humanity in action and people in tune with the needs of others…

If you've felt gratitude to someone unknown over the years, it might be nice to include them in your list of people who made a difference. It will also be a reminder that good people always exist in the world, even when the media tries to tell us otherwise.

Sharing the planet

For the first six years of my life, I shared the planet with Elvis Presley, Frank Sinatra, David Bowie and all four Beatles. They'd never heard of me, obviously, but I delight in the fact that, for those few years, we all existed in the world together, all sharing the same planet, living under the same sun. I didn't fully appreciate it at the time, of course, it's only now I look back and realise it feels significant to me as a music fan. And there are many other well-known names and faces from all walks of life who I feel privileged to have admired from afar as they went about the world spreading their talents, genius and wisdom…

In Section Five, we'll be looking at the people who have inspired you – past and present. But for now, as we're looking at the people who shared in the journey of your life, you might like to begin making a note of any famous faces who you feel glad to have been alive alongside. Choose from entertainers, sports people, authors, artists, politicians or royalty.

The chain

"Our history begins before we are born. We represent the hereditary influences of our race, and our ancestors virtually live in us."
James Nasmyth

Whether you've researched your family tree back to Doomsday, or only know the names of your grandparents, there is something thrilling about knowing we all come from a long line of ancestors. Especially if, like me, you love history. The thought that someone related to me may have seen Roman soldiers march by, or perhaps caught a small glimpse of a large Henry VIII blows my mind a little bit, I have to say. My attempts to trace my family tree didn't take me back that far, unfortunately, but my ancestors were alive in the world at the time – how exciting is that?!

These ancestors, however far removed they may be from us, are still part of our family, part of who we are, an unbreakable line continuing down the centuries. Their story is the prequel to our story, and it will continue long after we've reached our final chapter. How incredible, and what a privilege, to be a link in that chain.

A few years ago I began to trace my family tree. I knew I had Anglo-Indian ancestry on my Dad's side of the family, and a strong line of Londoners from my Mum's. But my searching also revealed links to South Shields and several generations of Geordies, as well as Dorset sail cloth weavers. What a colourful combination!

I'm not going to show you how to trace your family tree – there are plenty of organisations, websites, magazines, books etc. full of expertise and advice should you want it. But, to give you a heads-up, they will all suggest you start at the same place – by speaking to parents, grandparents and any other relations, who can share their knowledge of the family and, at the same time, give you an insight into their own life experience.

At the time of writing this, my Nanny Doris is in her 95th year. Doris is my maternal grandmother and from a family of Londoners – her father helped to build the underground and she lived through the blitz near Finsbury Park. I see her regularly and never tire of hearing her stories or run out of questions to ask her. She's getting frail but her mind, and memories, are sharp as a pin. When her time comes, I know I'll be so grateful to have shared those conversations with her. We share the same nose too…

If you have relations who can shine a light on your background story and are happy to share their memories, make the most of them. I can't tell you how many times I've sat down with bereaved families who have said "I wish I'd asked my dad more about his early life" or "I don't know the names of all the relatives in this photo – mum knew all of them but it's too late to ask now".

I'm all for living in the moment and appreciating the here and now, but we can still benefit from a step back in time. And give a nod to the future too, so, if you are enjoying this process of looking back on your life, there may be younger members of the family who would enjoy hearing about it. They are, after all, the next link in the chain – the keepers of the family flame. So keep sharing…

SECTION THREE
Memorable Moments

"I don't want to get to the end of my life and find that I lived just the length of it. I want to have lived the width of it aswell"
Diane Ackerman

So… you've drawn an outline of the journey of your life so far, and you've made a list of the people who accompanied you along the way. Now we're going to shine a light on the memorable moments during that journey – experiences that made you feel deliriously happy, moments when you were bursting with pride, and those challenging times when you may have hit rock bottom. These are the events that we remember most because they give meaning to our lives. All those dates, places and names would be just a black and white, one-dimensional list if these moments weren't there to add colour, drama and depth. They are the 'width' that Diane Ackerman refers to in her quote above – the icing, the cherry, the room with a view…

And whatever life you've lived, however quiet and uneventful you think your days have been, there will be plenty of stand-out experiences. You wouldn't believe the times I visit a bereaved family to talk about the life of their loved-one, and I'm met with the words "there isn't much to say really…" Then I find out their mum single-handedly raised ten children, won Miss Lovely Legs at Butlins, and survived two heart attacks. I wouldn't say that was an uneventful life, would you?

So prepare to become reaquainted with your own stand-out stories. Remember you made a start on thinking about memorable stories and anecdotes in Section One. And, like everything you've done so far, these stories will play a very useful part in our final section, when we pull everything together and look from your past to your future, and how you want to be remembered after you've gone.

Good times

"The moments of happiness we enjoy take us by surprise. It is not that we seize them, but that they seize us."
Ashley Montagu

I love the idea of being seized by happiness… don't you? And I'd like to think that we have all known (and continue to know) how that feels in life. From the thrill of a Christmas stocking at the end of our beds, to spontaneous evenings with mates, where our plans for "just the one drink…" lead to an unforgettable night of epic proportions. And what about the holidays? The family celebrations? The music festivals? The sporting triumphs?

And while happiness can be found in a single event, it can also be a stage in your life when things were going well – a job you had a passion for, a home you made your own, a special relationship, a summer of travel…

Look back through your life story, and the people you've known, and highlight when you were happiest, making a note of any particular events, anecdotes or stories. Try to include…

What happened and when?

Where were you?

Who were you with?

How did you feel?

Why was it so meaningful?

Proud Moments

"What would life be if we had no courage to attempt anything?"
Vincent Van Gogh

We all have reason to be proud of ourselves – whether we've reached the summit of Everest, or simply made it out of bed on a bad day. Pride comes in all shapes and sizes (and usually before a fall if you took advice from your parents)… But it's really important to recognise the moments in our lives when we think we did good. When we surpassed expectations, defied the odds, fulfilled a promise to ourselves, or made a difference to others.

Some of these proud moments will have been rewarded with trophies, qualifications, or pay rises. They may have resulted in new babies, smaller dress sizes or an 'all-clear' from the hospital. They may have been featured in the news, celebrated in the pub or simply gone unnoticed. But they still mattered… especially to you.

What have been your proudest moments so far? Have they been single events, such as running a marathon, or something longer term, like being a parent. Once again, use your life story and notes in previous sections to jog your memory. Think about …

Why was this a proud moment or aspect of your life?

What's the story behind it?

Where were you? How old were you? Who else was involved?

How did it make you feel?

Has it been recognised and remembered by others?

Challenging times

"Life's challenges are not supposed to paralyse you, they're supposed to help you discover who you are"
Bernice Johnson Reagon

Whatever challenges we face in life, we can guarantee there'll be a lesson for us in there somewhere – something to learn from once we emerge, dusting ourselves off from whatever struggle has come our way. The first lesson to learn is that every life has its share of struggles – sadly some more than others. But we all experience good times and bad times, ups and downs, gains and losses… it's what life is all about. And it's how we deal with these challenges that says the most about the people we are and what's important to us.

You may have had a difficult childhood, been divorced, unemployed, depressed. You may have experienced addiction, illness, fear, or loneliness. You will almost certainly have experienced loss, in some form, and bereavement. Or perhaps the challenge has been helping others in your life who have experienced some of the above.

It's really important to recognise these challenges in your life and see how they've played their part, alongside the good times and proud moments. In fact, you may find that these challenges also appear as proud moments, because you have come through a difficult time in your life, safe and sound, wiser than before and with a new outlook on the world. So, if you feel up to it, revisit some of those events and experiences that have been challenging, or perhaps reflect on just one. Make a note of…

What challenge(s) did you face?
How old were you?
How did it come about? Who else was involved?
How did it make you feel? How did you overcome it?
What did you learn from it?

Eventful lives

"And in the end it's not the years in your life that count… it's the life in your years"
Abraham Lincoln

If I had to choose one word that best describes how my work as a Celebrant makes me feel, I would say 'privileged'. To be entrusted with the telling of precious life stories, and what that life meant to others, is an absolute honour. Every story is unique and special in its own way, but some stories are, of course, more eventful than others…

In his early 20's Rav left Iran and moved to London to further his education and embrace a new life in England. And it was here that he met his wife Sandra. When they first married, nobody expected it to last. They were so different – in language, background, culture, religion – apparently they had nothing in common. The year after they married, they took an exciting road trip to Iran – travelling through Germany, Austria, Yugoslavia and Turkey. Once in Iran they visited Rav's family and Sandra was shown around his homeland, where they also had a second wedding ceremony.

Born in Poland in the late 1920's Marta's father was a high-ranking officer in the military and she and her siblings enjoyed a charmed life of wealth and privilege. The invasion of Poland during the Second World War would change all their lives forever. Taken prisoner and put onto cattle trucks heading for Siberia when she was 12, her family were forced to abandon their home, their belongings, and leave Poland with just the clothes they stood in. They lost everything. The indescribable horror of that time, experienced at such a tender age, formed the brave, strong, proud, fearless woman she would become.

Stuart's mum died of TB in her early 30's, and so, with his father away, 10-year-old Stuart and his brothers were placed in an orphanage. Here the boys were looked after and taught the skills they would need for life and employment. There is no doubt the boys would have missed their parents terribly, but a photograph of Stuart taken at the orphanage shows a grinning young lad in his shorts and blazer, with an arm around each of his brothers. At the age of 16, he joined the Royal Navy *as a boy bugler. He was then part of a ship's crew who went to the Far East to collect Japanese prisoners of war. Many of these brave men were too weak to survive the journey, so they were buried at sea, with Stuart playing the last post.*

SECTION FOUR
Music and Mementos

"A thing of beauty is a joy forever"
John Keats

Beauty comes in all forms, shapes and sizes. There is human beauty, natural beauty, artistic beauty. Beauty in words, music and objects. Beauty in gestures and actions. Beauty is everywhere, every day. Sometimes we just need to look a little harder for it. And alongside the beautiful, is the precious – the things that hold great meaning for us that we couldn't bear to part with.

You may have thought about, or been asked, the question "If there were a fire in your home, and your loved ones and pets were out safely, what would you try to save?" It's a tough one – do you think about what you might need on a practical level in the coming days? Do you try to grab the most expensive items? Or do you go for the items that hold the most meaning for you on a sentimental level – those things that may not be practical or valuable but are utterly priceless and irreplaceable to you?

In the section, we're going to look at three precious 'collections' that you may well decide to make a bee-line for in the event of such a catastrophe – music, photographs, and mementos. We'll look at how they fit into the story of your life, what they mean to you, where you keep them and who you share them with. Your answers will vary, of course, depending on your age. Your music collection, for example, may be vinyl, cassette, digital, or a combination of all of these. You may have original polaroid photographs from the 1970's or create polaroid-style images with a 21st century app on your smart phone. Perhaps you have bundles of hand-written letters or an answerphone message you'll never delete?

Previous sections will, again be useful, especially Section Three where we looked at significant and memorable moments. So enjoy another trip down memory lane…

The Soundtrack To Your Life

"Music is the emotional life of most people."
Leonard Cohen

People often ask me, "is it difficult to keep your own emotions under control when you're doing a funeral ceremony?" My answer – it usually depends what music has been chosen. Music is highly powerful and emotive, and once we've attached a song to a particular event in our lives or to someone special, it's virtually impossible to disconnect them. So if a family chooses a song that has emotional connections for me, I have to do all I can to distract my mind away from it. I'll form a detailed, mental shopping list, or think about what I'm cooking for tea, that sort of thing. I don't mean to be disrespectful to the family or deceased in question. But it's the only way to contain myself and keep it together. Of course, not all these songs are sad songs. Quite often there will be an up-beat piece of music that I find impossible to sit still to. But a dancing Celebrant would be just as bad as a crying one, so again, gentle foot taps are the order of the day…

• So what music is special to you?
• What have been the tracks of your years?
• Are there songs that remind you of meaningful times in your life, places, people, special events, good times?
• How about songs that helped you to face difficult moments, challenging events, break ups or break downs?
• Or songs that have no particular association but they just make you feel really good?
• Have you 'inherited' songs from loved ones. Are there songs you'd like to dedicate or hand-down to family and friends?

Add these songs to your life story, relationships, and special moments sections, and perhaps then make a playlist of your favourites. And even if you wouldn't describe yourself as a music fan, music will still have played a significant part in your life. You may not have been buying records or listening to the radio, but music still played its part in defining each decade you've lived through – whether that was the Big Band 40's, Swinging 60's or Electro 80's. So perhaps look at what you identified as your happiest times and see what music was hitting the airwaves.

This is your chance to take part in your very own Desert Island Discs, except you can choose as many songs as you like and I'll let you take them all with you!

What A Picture

"A photograph can be an instant of life captured for eternity that will never cease looking back at you."
Brigitte Bardot

Everywhere you look these days, people are 'capturing the moment'. Phones held aloft at music gigs and on the end of selfie sticks at tourist attractions. Wedding guests zooming in on the first dance while holiday makers immortalise the last sunset. Parents savouring baby's first steps, and pet owners capturing the four-legged funny bits. Everyone is clicking away and sharing in an instant.

I'm from a generation who takes pictures and videos on my phone but also remembers going on holiday with six rolls of film in her suitcase, returning home a week later to wait excitedly in Boots for the film to be developed. Oh the agony and the ecstasy of flicking through the prints to see what was in focus! Growing up in the 70's there are childhood polaroids of me in photo albums which my parents carefully tucked into plastic sleeves or stuck down with little gold-embossed corners. And very precious black and white photographs of my grandparents, equally treasured on the pages of albums or in frames on the wall.

Capturing the moment may seem to have become more important than the moment itself these days, but there is no denying the joy of a photograph and the memories that are encapsulated within its frame. Whether those images are on a flat screen or curling at the corners, they are precious to us, reminders of where we've been, who we've known, what we've seen, and, importantly, who we were in that moment.

• So what photographs do you have that hold meaning for you?
• Which ones reflect the journey of your life, the person you've been, the people you've known and loved, the adventures you've had, the proud moments you've been part of?
• Where are these photographs kept? Are any on display? Have you shared them with family and friends?
• And what photographs do you think really reflect the real you, as you see yourself? If you had to choose an image for the front of your 'order of service', which would it be?

Hidden Treasures

"Precious things are for those that can prize them."
Aesop's Fables

If asked what is the most valuable thing in life, I would say 'time', followed closely by 'health', as both are equally priceless and you don't really want one without the other. But I also appreciate this sense of priceless value can be applied to objects – the things we cherish for sentimental reasons that we can never bring ourselves to part with, no matter how many times we declutter, move house, or need to make room for newer, more practical things. These sentimental items could be letters, cards, newspaper cuttings, drawings, photographs, event tickets, cassette tapes, holiday souvenirs, video clips, clothing, autographs, jewellery, medals, menus… whatever we attach meaning to because they remind us of a person, a place, or a significant, memorable event in our lives.

These objects might be stored in a box under the bed or on display in your home. You might wear them every day, or appreciate their significance on anniversaries or special days of the year. However they are stored or used, they say something about what matters to you, why you wouldn't be without them, and why that fireman had to restrain you from running back into your burning home to retrieve them.

So what items do you treasure?
What's the story behind them?
How long have you had them?
Where are they kept and who else sees them?

Another very important question to ask yourself is - what will happen to these items when I am no longer here to appreciate their value?

There are some items - such as tickets or cards which hold great meaning to you which may not be so sentimental to others. But there will also be other items that you might want to pass on to specific family members or friends – a diamond ring, a Chanel handbag, a Gibson guitar, or a book of recipes, a first-edition LP, a small ornament with a special story. Again, write down your wishes - perhaps even little notes to go with each item. They will mean so much when the time comes.

SECTION FIVE

The Unique You

"Today you are you, that is truer than true. There is no-one alive who is you-er than you!"

Dr Seuss

We are all wonderfully unique, with our own special brand of magic that dazzles the world. We have our own personalities and characteristics, qualities and quirks, talents and skills, values and beliefs. We look different, sound different. And that's a truly beautiful thing. But it's a sad fact that in 2016 the tenth most googled question in the UK was "how to accept myself for who I am". That means there are a lot of people out there who are likely to be feeling unhappy, dissatisfied, and critical of themselves.

We should all – every single one of us – appreciate our uniqueness. We should take pride in it, cherish it… LOVE IT. We should recognise our value in the world and to others. Celebrate our differences. Be the best version of ourselves we can be. So that when we form relationships, it's the coming together of all these wonderful, unique lives – rather than feeling the need for us or others to conform to a 'type' or expecting others to come along and complete our lives for us. I don't mean that in an unromantic way – I'm all for falling in love and finding soul mates – but if we treat ourselves with respect, love and kindness, and recognise what makes us special, we are better equipped to deal with relationships, with the world around us, and harness our uniqueness in a positive way.

So, with that in mind, Section 5 is all about YOU. Because, while we've recognised the wonder of relationships and the meaning other people have brought to your lives so far, you could argue that the most important relationship we have in life is the one we have with ourselves. We'll look at what sets you apart, your personality and characteristics, where you values come from, your looks and mannerisms. How you see yourself, how others see you, and which unique individuals you have been inspired by.

Your Character and Qualities

When I meet bereaved families and we talk about their loved one's life and achievements, I always finish by asking "What were they like as a person?" It's a case of 'last but not least', because I believe it's the most important question – more important than where they went to school or what hobbies they had. But it's often the hardest question to answer. People can look blank or struggle to respond. So, without putting words into their mouths, I try to gently encourage them along, perhaps asking "Were they an outgoing sort of person or more reserved?", "were they creative" or "did they have a good sense of humour?" and gradually we build up a picture of this person they knew and loved. Such as…

Alan was thoroughly old-fashioned and very much set in his ways. All measurements had to be in centimetres and there was none of this small, medium, large nonsense. As for food, he knew what he liked, and he liked what he knew. Alan's horror following June's unsuccessful attempt to introduce garlic bread onto the menu one day, is a classic example. But he did love a cup of tea and was affectionately known to his family as 'tea belly'.

Now, none of us are saints – we all demonstrate a colourful mix of behaviours from the good, the bad and, at times, perhaps, even the ugly. And I believe it's important to give a full picture of who someone was, 'warts and all' as they say. But there are ways of being both accurate and respectful. For example, someone who was clearly argumentative, opinionated and brutally honest can be remembered as someone who 'knew their own mind and liked to share it'. And you can see that most family and friends who are gathered on the day will appreciate this refined honesty and welcome the opportunity to nod and smile because they recognise the person I'm talking about. And that's really important.

What's also important is recognising that how we see ourselves may be different from how others see us. For example, the person we are at home may be different to the person our colleagues see at work. So this is an opportunity for you to express what you think are the traits and qualities that define you.

SO… how would you describe your character, personality and qualities? Or perhaps choose five words you think describe you.
Do you strongly recognise any of these traits in your parents, grandparents or other family members?
Do you have children or grandchildren who have inherited these qualities from you?

Your Talents and Skills

"That's what I consider true generosity: you give your all, and yet you always feel as if it costs you nothing."
Simone De Beauvoir

Each and every one of us has a unique set of talents and skills. We are all good at something, and that something could be academic, artistic, practical, athletic, creative, humanitarian… or a combination of these. These talents may help you forge a successful career, benefit the community you live in, or the family you love. But each in its own way makes a difference – to us, to others and to the world in general.

What are your talents and skills?
How do you use them in life? (Look back at life story, achievements, proud moments etc. to remind you)
Do they make a difference to others?

Your Values and Beliefs

"To be yourself in a world that is constantly trying to make you something else is the greatest accomplishment."
Ralph Waldo Emmerson

With the exception of our unique genes, we all enter the world the same 'blank canvas'. In the years that follow we will be curious, impressionable, we'll learn from others and we'll learn for ourselves. And, before you know it, the things we do in life, the relationships we share, the places we visit, the events we experience, will all have played their part in making us who we are, shaping our outlook on the world and forming our values and beliefs.

What would you say your values are? Is kindness important? Fairness, compassion, empathy?

What matters to you? Is it success, happiness, your home, your family?

What issues do you care about? The environment, world peace, youth unemployment?

Do you have a faith or any spiritual beliefs?

Looks and Sounds

"Be yourself; everyone else is already taken."
Oscar Wilde

We've looked at all your personality traits, attributes, talents and values, but what about the most obvious aspects of what makes you unique – how you look and sound? I absolutely love that fact that as humans we come in all shapes and sizes, shades and styles. Just take a moment, next time you are out and about, and look at everyone around you. Such an incredible mix of heights and hair colours, face shapes and distinguishable features, ways of walking and talking.

I think it's sad that so many people, especially women, seem to feel dissatisfied with how they look, believing they must conform to a certain shape (usually thin) or age (very young), even going so far as to having bits cut off or filled out. Yes, we'd all like to feel attractive, perhaps lose a few pounds here and there. But we all might feel happier in our own skins if we celebrated differences a little more, saw the beauty in them, appreciated what our bodies actually do for us rather than how they look to others. It's a privilege to grow older so don't we owe it to ourselves to do those things?

- You have your own personal look – for example, are you tall? Are your fingers long? Your eyes wide?
- How do you like to dress? What's your style? Has this changed over the years?
- What do you sound like? Do you have a regional accent? Are you softly spoken? A fast talker? What sayings do you use?
- Who do you look and sound like in your family? Are these living relatives or ancestors?
- Are there any quirks or distinguishing characteristics that are unique to you? A dimple when you smile or a booming laugh?

Lasting Impressions

You may have read through this section, asking you to identify your qualities, skills and characteristics and thought – "don't ask me!" Which is fair enough. You may feel others have a better idea of what you're good at and how you come across. But are you brave enough to ask them? If so, go ahead! But remember, unless you approach family, friends and colleagues who 'know their own mind and like to share it' you may not get a completely full picture. And, likewise, if you do ask someone who is brutally honest, you might not want to hear their verdict!

If you don't feel up to the face-to-face approach, other places to look for comments on your character, skills etc. over the years are school reports, written feedback from employers, 'thank you' cards… if you've kept them, that is. Apparently my history teacher believed I was "A pleasure to teach with a very high standard of work." My Chemistry teacher, however, felt I had "lost interest and therefore underachieved." Oh well… you can't be good at everything can you?

Inspirations

In Section Two – Your Relationships – you began to make of list of any famous faces you feel glad to have shared the planet with. Now that you've examined more closely your own skills, values and qualities, take another look at that list and think again about who has inspired you in life. Which artists, musicians, campaigners, scientists, politicians, humanitarians, adventurers, athletes, historical figures have helped to form your view of the world, given you words of wisdom, new ways of thinking, brave ideas, shaped your tastes and preferences, touched your soul, rocked your world?

SECTION SIX
Onward Journeys

"I don't know whether you can look at your past and find, woven like the hidden symbols on a treasure map, the path that will point to your final destination"
Jodi Picoult

There is no denying that our past shapes us – it makes us the people we are, forms our views on the world and teaches us valuable lessons. It provides a multitude of experiences, events, achievements, relationships, journeys and memories – our very own multi-coloured, super-sensory, wide-screened epic production starring… drumroll… us!

Throughout Part One you've journeyed into your past, shining a spotlight on yourself at various stages and ages, re-visiting significant places, hearing old, familiar tunes, becoming reaquainted with friends and relations, and, I hope, uncovering some forgotten treasures. So before we jump across to Part Two of Remember Me, and look at how all this information can be used in your own life celebration ceremony, it's important to just pause here a moment – to think about how this experience has made you feel, what it's revealed to you about your life so far, and were there clues to how you'd like that life journey to continue? Because I hope you all have many years ahead of you to enjoy, before that life is commemorated.

So in this final section, we're going to take stock – we'll go through what you uncovered about your life so far, the highs, lows, and lessons learnt. Then we'll give some thought to what may have been missing – the things you haven't done, experienced or expressed - as well as the things you want to do more of, or enjoy again. We'll come up with some future goals, ideas for sharing your life lessons and perhaps write your own manifesto. Finally, some positive thoughts to see you on your way as you embark on the next stage of your life story, and prepare to take the brave step of looking at your own life celebration and the legacy you want to leave behind.

Taking Stock

However long you've spent on Part One, whatever format you've compiled information in, and however much you've contributed, you will, I hope, have something to look back on now. Because, as well as being a wonderful collection of stories, memories and mementos encapsulating you and your life that can be shared with your loved-ones as well as form part of your life celebration ceremony, you also have at your fingertips the clues to what will make you happy in the future – what will continue to give your life meaning, the direction you want to head in, and some priorities to take forward, so you can make the most of the time you have to come.

So I suggest you return to each section you've completed and, as you look through, remind yourself of the following...

Happy Times

- When were you happiest? What made you happy at this point?
- What were you doing? Who were you with?
- What reminders do you have of them?

Difficult Times

- When were the low points? What happened?
- Why were they difficult? Who else was involved?
- What changed?

Proudest Moments

- What have you been most proud of? Were these moments shared with others?
- What made them so significant and meaningful to you?
- What reminders do you have of them?

You At Your Best

When would you say you were at your best in terms of what was happening in your life, what you were doing, how you behaved, how you felt, how you looked, what you believed in at the time and valued most?

Using your answers to Happy Times, Difficult Times, Proudest Moment and You At Your Best, you can identify where your life's highs and lows have been, what went right, what went wrong, the unexpected curveballs thrown, the strokes of luck, the good, the bad, the beautiful… and how you faced up to it all.

Be sure to highlight – big and bold – those answers because, frankly, this information is gold dust. Having sifted through the years you're left with these valuable nuggets that not only keep you rich in happy and proud moments, they are also a measure of what matters to you, lessons in avoiding the pitfalls that snagged you before, and reminders of how to stay true to your authentic self. So let's look at how you use this information going forward…

Where Next?

"Only put off until tomorrow what you are willing to die having left undone."
Pablo Picasso

As well as wanting to use my skills and experience to help you have a meaningful funeral ceremony, my inspiration for putting together Remember Me also came from a genuine desire for people to feel good about who they are, their unique place in the world, the lives they have lived, and their lives to come. And, now you've reflected on your life so far, we can ask that all-important question… what do you want to do with the rest of your life?

More of the good stuff

The answer is pretty obvious isn't it? You know what's made you happy in the past, what's inspired you, who you've enjoyed being with. Why not do more of the same? Well, I appreciate it may not be as simple as that. If you were happiest as a carefree 17-year-old backpacking around the world with your mates, and now you have a job to do, a mortgage to pay and family to look after, that might not be so easy to plan. Anyway, you may be perfectly happy with your life as it is and not looking to 'recreate' moments from the past.

BUT you can acknowledge what it was about those happy moments that had such a positive impact on you. And, if those things, ie. discovering new places, taking time out, feeling the sun on your back, spending time with friends… still resonate with you, think of achievable ways to incorporate them into your current life on a more regular basis.

Playing to your strengths

You've thought about your talents and skill, your qualities and characteristics, your values and beliefs… are they being put to good use? Look back at Section Five and remind yourself what makes you… you? What are your strengths? What sets you apart? Are talents being wasted? Beliefs being compromised? Beauty being hidden?

What's missing?

For some, the answer to a happier and more fulfilling life may not lie in what's happened to you already. It may, actually, be found in what hasn't happened to you at all… yet. There may be things you haven't done but are longing to do, things you want to experience or express that just haven't been realised or come to fruition. There may have been missed opportunities, wrong circumstances, or, quite simply, the time wasn't quite right. Now it is… or it soon will be.

Seize the day... or simply enjoy it

"You don't get to choose how you're going to die. Or when. You can only decide how you're going to live. Now."
Joan Baez

When you looked back on your life, saw photographs of yourself from years gone by, did you think "where has the time gone?" Well, time has a habit of going by, and it appears to speed up the older you get! When I was young I remember being impatient – wishing I was a teenager when I was still in single figures, wishing I was working when I was still at school, wishing for Christmas again when the decorations had barely been put back in the loft. My mum always said the same thing to me "Nicola, don't wish your life away". And she was right.

Life is so precious, and it's precious because, at some point unknown to us, it ends. So life needs to be savoured, appreciated, enjoyed, and lived. As the artist Francis Bacon said "Begin doing what you want to do now.We are not living in eternity. We have only this moment, sparkling like a star in our hand and melting like a snowflake."

If you've decided to do more of the things that make you happy, then plan them in. But be realistic about what you can do and when. 'Seize The Day' doesn't mean fitting all your dreams and goals into the next 24 hours. Just make small steps towards them, and each step should, eventually, get you where you want to go. But remember there is no right or wrong direction to head to from here. In fact, you don't have to head anywhere at all. Looking back on your life can simply be an interesting interlude – a pause for thought. And that's absolutely fine.

Passing on Your Wisdom

"Knowing yourself is the beginning of all wisdom"
Aristotle

The one thing you can guarantee in life is that you never stop learning. Whether it's from the experiences of others or your own mistakes, there are lessons for us right up until our last breath. And that's a good thing. It's what makes our journey so interesting, and also allows us to have an impact on the lives of others and on the world itself. Hopefully, in a positive way.

You have lived and learned. All being well, you will continue to do so for many more years. And that means you know a lot... you really do. You have a vast, rich, interesting, colourful store of information and experiences that will be useful to others. Whether that knowledge includes initiatives for world peace, or baking the perfect sponge cake, you can contribute to the well-being of others in some way. So think about how your knowledge and experience may benefit others. This could simply be within your own familiar circle of family and friends, or out in to the wider world.

You may also want to come up with your own manifesto based on, not only your knowledge and experience, but also what matters to you. Something that reflects your values and beliefs. If you feel strongly about something, put it out there (you'll see my own Manifesto on my website). Your voice is as valuable as anyone else's and there are more platforms than ever to speak out from.

Conclusion

However much of Part One you've completed, you have taken the time to think about who you are, where you've come from and why you and your life matter. So if this experience has left you feeling good about yourself and your place in the world, and given you some ideas for the future, then that's just great. In fact it's better than great – it's fantastic! I appreciate that recalling past events, looking at old photographs, hearing emotive songs, may have stirred some strong emotions at times. But hopefully, the overwhelming feeling is a positive one.

You may have ended up with a wonderful digital edition of your life story that you can share with the world. Or you may have a little notebook or memory box that will now be tucked away for safekeeping. What you now choose to do with all this information is entirely up to you. Whatever form your life story and notes have taken, and however private you want them to be for now, I would suggest that you let your loved ones know that, somewhere safe, you have this information. And, if you are happy for all, or some of it, to be put towards a celebration of your life after you've gone*, then Part Two awaits you…

* You may not want to wait until you are gone for a celebration of your life to take place. You may want to throw a party and celebrate while you are still here! And why not? Although if you are in good health and your party doesn't fall on your birthday, you may need to do some explaining. But that's OK. Just tell your guests "I'm celebrating my life and everyone who has played a part in it". Then all you need to do is have a night to remember…

5 REMEMBER ME
PART TWO: YOUR CEREMONY

Welcome to Part Two – and well done for taking the brave and positive step of thinking about your farewell wishes. Over six different stages we'll take a deeper look in to what makes a meaningful life celebration and your options for the type of funeral ceremony you feel would mean something to you and your loved ones.

Along the way we'll look at everything from flowers and coffins, to music and photographs, together with the all-important story of your life, personal messages and other meaningful words, plus advice on how to share your wishes with your loved ones.

Part Two combines all the information and thoughts you gathered in Part One, together with my knowledge and experience of the funeral profession and creating life-led ceremonies. It won't be morbid – I promise! Here's what we'll be covering...

ONE: THE F-WORD

We'll start with a reminder of three very good reasons why you should think about your funeral ceremony, and what a funeral is really for.

TWO: TYPES OF FUNERAL CEREMONY

This section covers the all-important question of Burial or Cremation and the considerations that may have an impact on your decision. Plus the options and possibilities for where and how you'd like to be laid to rest, and the style of ceremony that is best suited to your wishes and beliefs.

THREE: YOUR CEREMONY

We begin to look at the many ways you can create a ceremony that is uniquely personal to you, starting with choices such as style of coffin, how you'd like to be dressed, the wonderful, colourful world of floral tributes, and memorable ways to arrive on the day itself.

FOUR: MUSIC AND IMAGES

Music plays an essential part in any funeral ceremony, reflecting your tastes and personality, as well as the feelings you have for life and your loved ones. So how do you choose music and at what point in the ceremony is it played? We also look at the use of photographs and video/audio recordings.

FIVE: MEANINGFUL WORDS

What will be said when everyone gathers to say farewell to you? How can your life story, your qualities and characteristics, your achievements and feelings be shared in an accurate and meaningful way? We answer all these questions, together with thoughts on poems and readings, and sharing personal messages.

SIX : FINAL THOUGHTS

In our final part we discuss how you can live on through charitable donations and gifts, and the comfort your loved ones will gain from gathering together after the ceremony to share memories and raise a glass to you.

First a reminder on capturing information...

The desired outcomes of completing this Part Two section are, first of all, getting down all your thoughts, ideas and wishes regarding your funeral ceremony, and, secondly, being able to pass on that precious information to those who will need it. You may wish to make your ideas known to your loved ones as soon as you've compiled them (or even share them as you go along) or place your wishes somewhere they can be found when the time comes. We covered the subject of how you capture this information at the start of Part One, so you may simply wish to continue with whatever format you began with then. Or you may want to try something different. Here's a reminder of your options…

Digital
Type up your wishes – so you can easily add to or amend things when you want to. You can also get as creative, designing your ideas, adding images, links etc. And when you're done you can save the document to your desk-top or tuck it in a folder somewhere. Just make sure your loved ones know it exists and it can be found when needed.

Get Creative
If you have artistic talents you may prefer to collate your farewell wishes in a more visual and creative way then. Drawings, illustrations, photographs, scrap books… They will make a lovely memento for those closest to you. Just remember, the same 'rules' apply – are your wishes clear, do your loved one's know they exist and where to find them?

Hand-written

"The beauty and nobility, the august mission and destiny, of human handwriting."

George Bernard Shaw, Pygmalion

Every now and again, families show me hand-written lists of music, poems, even final letters, from their loved ones. And just seeing the unique, personal handwriting of someone whose life I'll be giving thanks for, gives me a meaningful connection to them – even more so than seeing their photograph. Some of these precious bits of paper I'm given are used envelopes, shopping lists, even betting slips! But you might want to get yourself a nice notebook instead.

Once again, make sure your family/friends know it exists and where you keep it. And if you are known for having, let's say, an 'interesting' handwriting style, remember it needs to be legible for others!

Audio and Video

You might want to mix it up and combine typed or written notes with a recording. Certainly hearing the voice of someone dearly departed, or seeing their face in front of you once again, is a gift technology has made possible for everyone. But remember too that if this is a 'surprise' you are leaving for people after you've gone, it is going to be hugely emotional, both for you to record and, especially, for them to experience. So that does add a whole new layer of meaning to what you choose to say.

SECTION ONE
The F-Word

Why Should I Think About My Funeral Ceremony?

We've covered the benefits of planning and talking about your funeral in previous chapters but, If you are still in any doubt about it, here is a reminder…

1. One day you won't be here any more and those closest to you will be trying to come to terms with that heart-breaking event, while at the same time being asked to make all sorts of decisions and answer questions like 'did your mum want to be buried or cremated?' If you can at least give your loved ones some clues before you go, it will make a huge difference to how they cope with all this.

2. Your family will, of course, want to make their own contributions to proceedings – this is the last thing they can do for you, so, it's incredibly important that they are given the opportunity to express how they feel about you and your life. BUT, when all is said and done, it was indeed your life. And no-one knows your life better than you. So as others give their own perspective on who you were, what you've done, and what it meant to them, how about sharing what it meant to you and making a few contributions of your own?

3. Thinking about your own funeral ceremony can have a positive effect on how you view your life. Yes really! The idea of it may seem depressing at first, but acknowledging your mortality can give a meaningful perspective on your life and what you choose to do with the time you have. Life is precious and finite, it helps to be reminded of that.

What's A Funeral Ceremony For?

"Everything that has a beginning has an ending. Make your peace with that and all will be well."
Buddhist Saying

Choices… Choices… That's the beauty of funerals these days. You can decide, among other things, the type of ceremony you'd like, where it's held, who conducts it, how you arrive, what music is played, what is said… you can even decide not to have one at all.

But for most of us, a funeral ceremony provides an opportunity to give thanks for a person's life, to express our feelings of love and affection for them, to celebrate and pay tribute to all they achieved, enjoyed and experienced while they were here, to share memories, to comfort each other, and, of course, to say farewell. And if you are able to play a part in the creation and content of your own funeral ceremony, then it will be even more personal and meaningful for everyone involved.

You can think about and decide on as much or as little of your funeral ceremony as you like. And while this isn't a definitive guide to the world of funerals, if there is something you'd like to request or comment on that hasn't been covered, including end of life issues, such as how you'd like to be cared for should you become terminally ill, then add it to your wishes.

Funeral Directors

If you want the services of a funeral director, and have a preference in terms of which firm is used to take care of you and your family, then include their name in your wishes. If you don't have a firm in mind, but would like to specify one, ask for recommendations from family and friends who may have required the services of a funeral director within the last 12 months. It's best to have current recommendations as, like all businesses, funeral directors can change hands or staff. You will have a choice of independent, family-run funeral directors, together with funeral homes belonging to chains, such as Co-op Funeralcare. I'm only familiar with the funeral directors in my own area, so it's not fitting for me to make recommendations to you. But the most important requirement is that they come across as both caring and professional, they listen to your needs and provide information without the 'hard sell'. You can always contact local funeral homes yourself – perhaps even pop in next time you're in town. Don't worry – you're not tempting fate – just being organised!

SECTION TWO

Types of Funeral Ceremony

The Big Questions – Burial or Cremation?

If you only want to make one decision about your funeral ceremony, this is the one – do you want to be buried or cremated? It's important that you express this wish beforehand so your family aren't left with an agonising choice, wondering which you would have preferred. The outcome of your decision will also have an impact on where your funeral ceremony takes place, in particular the committal aspect of it (the 'farewell' part of a ceremony where you are lowered into the ground at burial or committed for cremation). Here are some considerations to help you…

Burial

"To lie in the soft brown earth, with the grass waving above one's head, and listen to silence. To have no yesterday and no tomorrow. To forget time, to forgive life, to be at peace."
Oscar Wilde

Is there a specific place where you'd like to be buried? A local cemetery, church graveyard, or Green Burial site? Contrary to popular belief, you can be buried in your own back garden, but it does, of course, require the fulfilment of certain conditions, such as inclusion on the house deeds (not to mention the agreement of your loved ones who will be gardening, and BBQ-ing next to you for however many years, or may want to sell the house at some point). The same goes for any burial plot – permissions need to be given and conditions met. There's also cost to consider – burial is almost always more expensive than cremation, as it involves purchasing a plot, as well as a burial fee, grave digging costs, a possible headstone, etc. And if you want to be buried in an area where you are no longer a resident, the fees will rise astronomically.

In terms of the ceremony, you can have a graveside service, although the unpredictable British weather can make for interesting proceedings! It's one thing standing in a summer meadow, sharing memories as the sun shines and birds sing, but quite another when the wind is howling and I'm shouting to be heard over the drumming of rain on umbrellas. Some cemeteries, however, have a chapel where you can hold a ceremony first before making your way to the graveside for the committal. Although some of these chapels are very small, not particularly comfortable, and audio-visual facilities virtually non-existent. There's also the option of a church service, if you are religious. Or you could have your ceremony at a separate venue either before or after the burial, such as a village hall, function room, even your own home, where refreshments can also be taken there afterwards.

Just remember, if you wish to be 'present' at your own ceremony, the venue will need to be happy with a coffin on the premises and considerations made if there are steep stairs or anything that might prove hazardous to your arrival. You don't want to make too much of a dramatic entrance…

Cremation

All towns and cities will have a local crematorium. You may have a preference about which one you'd like to be taken to, but do consider where your loved ones and friends will be travelling from to get there on the day. The crematorium will have one or two chapels where the funeral ceremony and committal can be held together. You may even wish to have your ashes scattered or interred in the grounds of the crematorium a few days later, in which case you can do everything in one place. How convenient!

However, sometimes people choose to simply have a committal at the crematorium, with or without loved ones present. Then, as we discussed for burials, you could have a separate ceremony at another venue either before or after the committal. We'll talk more about alternative venues later…

Crematorium services do have time restrictions. For example, my local crematorium has 30 minute services – this includes the time it takes to enter and leave the chapel so you actually end up with about 20 minutes for the ceremony itself, although you can book an extended ceremony of 60 minutes. Other crematoriums have 45 minutes or services on the hour. Fees vary depending on whether you are having just a committal, a standard ceremony or extended ceremony. The time of day can also factor in the price – early services tend to be cheaper, while a Saturday ceremony will be much more expensive.

Most, if not all, crematoriums are happy to show people around, with prior arrangement. It's certainly worth doing as, not only do you get to see the chapels and grounds, but you'll also be given a glimpse of what happens behind the scenes. This is all done very sensitively, of course, and it gives the general public a chance to learn about what really happens and reassuringly puts to rest some of the myths and misinformation that seems to abound, ie. that coffins are re-used afterwards, or that ashes from various bodies are combined. Neither is true!

The Weird and Wonderful

There are some interesting (and downright bizarre) developments happening in the world of funerals, in particular the options for what we can do with our bodies, from freeze drying and mushroom suits, to eternal reefs and space burial. Some of them are available now, some are still being fine-tuned. Who knows what will be on offer when our time comes?! But if you've seen something that takes your fancy, write it down. You might also want to start saving as most come with a hefty price tag!

Your Ashes

"To live in this world you must be able to do three things: to love what is mortal; to hold it against your bones knowing your own life depends on it; and, when the time comes to let it go, to let it go."
Mary Oliver

With a cremation you do, of course, have cremated remains to consider. Ashes are available for collection a certain number of days after the funeral, either by the Funeral Directors on behalf of your family, or by your family. This will have been agreed beforehand. Or, as I mentioned earlier, your ashes can remain at the crematorium and be scattered or interred there by staff alone, by staff together with family members, or in a short ceremony with a Celebrant or minister.

If you don't want your final resting place to be the grounds of a crematorium then, frankly, the world is your oyster! Is there a favourite spot where you'd like to have your ashes scattered – a beach, a garden, by rocket into the sky? Or would you like your ashes interred alongside a loved one in a cemetery or underneath a tree in a Woodland Burial Ground? Or perhaps you'd be happier in a nice urn on the mantlepiece where you can still see the telly? The decision is yours. Although, like most things we've talked about so far, there can be considerations and permissions to factor in – requesting your ashes are scattered in your favourite pub, for example, might not go down well with the landlord and locals. So check first.

Memorial Ceremonies

We've talked about funeral ceremonies which happen on the same day as the committal – either at the same time, beforehand or afterwards. But if you want more of a celebration of life, or memorial ceremony, on another day, away from the committal, you perhaps have more freedom of venue and location. You'll notice this often happens for public figures or celebrities, where there is a private family funeral but friends and colleagues gather for a memorial ceremony in the weeks that follow. So you could have a special gathering somewhere much more personal to you – on a beach where you holidayed, in a park where you walked the dog, a pub that was your favourite watering hole or some other landmark which has meaning to you and your loved ones. These provide the opportunity for more of a 'party' in your honour, if that takes your fancy. It could also tie in with the scattering of your ashes.

What If There Is No Body To Bury Or Cremate?

This might happen if someone has left their body to medical science, chosen to end their life at a facility such as Dignitas, or perhaps their body was never recovered following an accident. But in all these cases, and others, you can still have a memorial ceremony. I did such a ceremony for a man who was lost at sea and it was a truly wonderful event, in terms of being both comforting and uplifting. It gave his family and friends the much-needed opportunity to come together, acknowledge his loss, celebrate his life and say farewell in their own way.

What Do You Want The Focus Of Your Ceremony To Be?

Funeral ceremonies aren't neatly divided into the religious and the non-religious. That's a good thing, as far as I can see because we're all uniquely different and each funeral ceremony should reflect that. I approach each of my ceremonies with the intention of capturing the essence of the person who has died – their character and qualities, their individual beliefs, values and wishes – while reflecting the wishes and feelings of their family. But for the purposes of helping you decide what sort of ceremony you might like, and the type of person who could lead that ceremony, I will 'categorise' your main options. Just keep in mind how you'd like people to feel on the day, as well as what fits with your idea of giving thanks for a life…

A 'Life-Led' Ceremony

"We all die. The goal isn't to live forever, the goal is to create something that will."
Chuck Palahniuk

This is a funeral ceremony where you, your life, and the people who shared your life, are the main focus of events. You can make this as colourful as you like with all sorts of music, video clips, tributes, photographs. Or it can be a simple, un-fussy affair.

Whatever you decide, this would be led by a Funeral Celebrant, like me, (also known as Civil Celebrants or Independent Celebrants) or a Humanist Celebrant. You could choose your own Celebrant, even go so far as to plan your ceremony with one beforehand should you wish to. But bear in mind that if you plan your ceremony now while you are, hopefully, in good health, you may outlive the Celebrant who could retire (or even expire!) before you need them.

Whoever you, or your family choose, the Celebrant needs to be a good listener – absolutely in tune with your needs – they must be able to write a good ceremony which is as comforting as it is meaningfully 'enjoyable', and deliver it in a warm, professional manner. They will also be responsible for setting the right tone on the day so it's important to choose someone who can do all these things in keeping with your wishes. A tall order and, needless to say, some Celebrants are better than others, so get recommendations from people you know, as well as those in the funeral world – crematorium staff see a wide range of Celebrants every week so they are good people to ask.

Your ceremony could also be led by members of your own family or friends, which would make things very personal indeed. Although it may still be wise to have a Celebrant to simply act as a 'master of ceremonies' to make introductions and guide things along. It's not easy to organise things and deal with practicalities on the day when emotions are running high.

A 'Life-Led' Ceremony With Some Spiritual or Religious Content

The same as a life-led ceremony but with the addition of a little bit of spiritual content such as a hymn or religious reading. This could be anything from The Lord's Prayer to Buddhist teachings. Or you may just want to have a hymn as it reminds you of school, your wedding, or because you simply like the tune. People also choose hymns because they have family members who are religious or would appreciate the opportunity to sing together. A Celebrant can still perform this type of ceremony – the religious or spiritual aspects are read on your behalf rather than coming from any beliefs the Celebrant may or may not have. Humanist Celebrants have a non-religious philosophy and have, traditionally, been against performing this type of ceremony.

A Fully Religious Ceremony

"I am ready to meet my Maker. Whether my Maker is prepared for the great ordeal of meeting me is another matter"
Winston Churchill

If you have a strong faith or are a regular church-goer you will, no doubt, desire a fully religious ceremony led by a minister or relevant faith leader. You can specify who you'd like but, again, depending on the time between your planning and passing, it may not be possible.

A word about fees…
Whoever takes your ceremony will charge for their services. These vary from Celebrant to Celebrant and, of course, there are also church and ministers fees. These fees change annually but if you want an indication of costs, you will be able to look on-line or you can ask your local funeral director.

SECTION THREE
Your Ceremony

"To thine own self be true"
Shakespeare

This is the part where you can really make your mark on proceedings and help to create a funeral that is uniquely personal to you. It could simply be choosing your favourite flower or a poem, or, later, going as far as writing your own life story and recording a video message for everyone so you can actually be seen and heard on the day. It's really up to you how much or how little you want to be involved. And, of course, you can start to use the information you gathered together in Part One of the course – for example, your interests may dictate the style of vehicle you arrive in, or your unique style may influence how you want to be dressed. And don't forget these farewell wishes of yours can be changed or added to at any time.

Choosing A Coffin

You won't believe how many different types of coffin are now available, both in terms of materials used, their shape and colour, not to mention cost. From your traditional wooden coffins to hand-painted caskets, from sheep's wool or woven banana leaf, to coffins shaped liked aeroplanes or canal boats. I've seen all sorts of lovely personalised coffins over the years with pictures of butterflies, steam trains, football shields and lavender fields. There have been beautiful willow caskets interwoven with wild flowers for natural burials, and cosy woollen coffins. And, perhaps most touching, cardboard coffins decorated by the family, with children's painted handprints, photographs stuck on, glitter, stickers and hand-written messages of love.

You may feel coffins are a waste of money, considering what ultimately happens to them, and choose the most basic and inexpensive model available. That makes perfect sense, but if you think you'd like to make a more colourful statement when you arrive for your final farewell… go for it. It's a very personal choice– and the choice is, as I said, wide and varied – so rather than me recommend any particular manufacturers, have a browse online to see what's currently available.

Favourite Flowers

"Flowers are a proud assertion that a ray of beauty out values all the utilities of the world."
Ralph Waldo Emmerson

Like coffins, floral tributes come in all sorts of wonderful shapes, sizes and designs these days. From your traditional casket display and individual letters, to baskets of fruits and veg, pints of Guinness and snooker tables! But I think the nicest floral tribute I've seen was a simple bunch of flowers cut from the lady's garden that very morning by her children and tied with a yellow ribbon. You may have a favourite flower, a meaningful colour you'd like represented, a seasonal display, or flowers and plants which reflect a favourite holiday destination or where you were born, such as Scottish thistles. You may want to cheer everyone up with big, yellow sunflower heads. Or, perhaps, letting your loved ones decide could be their way of 'saying it with flowers'…

What Do You Want To Be Dressed In?

"You never realise how much of your background is sewn into the lining of your clothes."
Tom Wolfe

Do you have a favourite dress? A cup-winning football shirt? A shade of lipstick you're never without? If so, and you'd like to be wearing them as you are laid to rest, make a note of it. Families I meet do often tell me they've chosen something special for their loved ones – 'mum has her favourite scarf' or 'dad's wearing his best tie'. We've even had Santa socks and gardening gloves! There are, however, crematorium guidelines regarding clothing and coffin content in order to minimise air pollutants, ie. clothing should be of natural fibres, no PVC, glass or plastic. There will also be regulations for natural burial grounds. But, those aside, there is still plenty of scope for personal touches.

Making An Entrance

Would you be happy to arrive at your ceremony in a beautifully polished hearse or would you like to consider another choice of vehicle? You could have a motorbike, a horse and carriage, a flatbed truck or a tractor. If you served in the Armed Forces you could have a flag bearer from the Royal British Legion or representatives from your regiment as a 'guard of honour'. I've seen some wonderful welcomes for people, from Scooter Club mates revving their Vespas and Lambrettas, to New Orleans-style jazz bands and the haunting sound of a lone piper. All of these 'entrances' helped to set a special tone for the ceremony and give it an individual feel from the very start.

Crowd Control

Do you have any thoughts on who you might like to 'invite' to your ceremony? Just so you know, you can't actually prevent anyone from attending your funeral ceremony if it's in a crematorium chapel or church, as they are seen as public events. Private ceremonies are another matter. But would you prefer a small gathering of immediate family and close friends, or would you like to know that anyone who ever knew you – from school friends and work colleagues, to fellow club members and pub regulars – were gathered to see you off? Obviously a lot of this depends on when your time comes, who you still know and if you've outlived others, but you might like to set out your preferences now. If you have contact numbers for any of these people then put them together with your wishes so you family can get in touch. If they are no longer in your area, then they won't see any announcement in the paper, should you have one.

SECTION FOUR
Music and Images

Meaningful Music

"After silence, that which comes nearest to expressing the inexpressible is music."

Aldous Huxley

Music has the power to move us… and never more so than at a funeral ceremony, where song choices have a strong, emotional impact on people, not just in terms of tearfulness but also the ability to create feelings of joy, comfort, nostalgia, as well as reflecting a person's character, interests or talents. I did a ceremony once for a ballroom dancer – his black patent dance shoes sat on top of the coffin – and when we played a waltz half-way through the ceremony his friends spontaneously partnered up and began dancing around the room. That was beautiful. As were the tears of laughter when people asked for 'Let's Do It' by Victoria Wood or clapping along to 'Happy' by Pharrell Williams. There has also been live music – choirs performing for fellow singers, grandchildren playing assorted instruments for Nanny or Granddad, even a ukulele band with a rousing rendition of 'You Are My Sunshine'.

Music really sets the tone for the ceremony, especially as it's the first thing people hear as they enter, and it will make all the difference to how they feel when the ceremony ends and they return to their own lives. Music choices are usually made based on one of the following reasons; it was a favourite tune of the person who's died, the sentiment of the song reflects how their loved ones are feeling, the lyrics have a fitting message and significance, or the song will cheer everyone up, make them smile and laugh. Whatever the reason, as long as the song has some sort of meaning to you or your loved ones. and not about what others 'expect' to hear, or what you think 'should' be played, that's all that matters.

In terms of when they are played, it's nice to have something to accompany you, your family and friends into the venue at the beginning, one or two songs to listen to during the ceremony itself – giving everyone an opportunity to sit and think about you – and something to see everyone out at the end (the cheerier the better). I've facilitated many a sing-a-long at the end of ceremonies, from 'We'll Meet Again' to football anthems or 'Bring Me Sunshine' made famous by Morecambe and Wise. So it's not just hymns that allow people to sing together. And these sing-a-longs, together with other upbeat tunes, mean people take their leave of you with a smile.

We've already looked at music, of course, in Part One - Your Life. So you can use the information from 'The Soundtrack To Your Life' to help you choose the music you want people to hear on the day. Songs performed, perhaps, by a favourite singer, or capturing the special times in your life. Are there lyrics among those songs that reflect how you feel about your life and your loved ones? Do you want people to tap their feet, sing along, or even dance their way out of the room? Whatever your thoughts on music, even if you only choose one song by way of contribution… just knowing it was your choice will make all the difference on the day, and allow your loved ones to choose the songs that remind them of you, and what you meant to them.

Just a word of advice though – make sure your music choices are actually available. For example, if you went to see your favourite band in concert and request a song to be played specifically from that event, unless it was recorded on the night and released as an official recording, you won't get your wish The same goes for Youtube clips. So do check before you make specific requests, or alternatively leave a bit of wriggle room so your loved-ones can come up with the next best thing.

Photographs and Video

"One day your life will flash before your eyes. Make sure it's worth watching."
Anon.

The funeral industry is slowly making friends with modern technology, and that's a good thing in terms of having more personalised ceremonies. In addition to original recordings of music played through speakers during services (as opposed to an organist sitting at the back) many crematoriums also have large screens which provide an opportunity for photographic slide shows or video footage.

We've just talked about the impact of music on the day, but if you put music together with images you really do have a powerful combination. Some families produce their own presentations which are then downloaded, while others send individual photographs to the crematorium music providers in the order they want them and their music choice is fitted alongside – the time each picture remains on the screen is worked out based on the song length. Be aware that while music is included in the standard crematorium fee, slideshows or video will be extra. You can also pay to have your ceremony recorded onto a CD or filmed via webcast on the day. All these options relate to crematorium ceremonies where the audio-visual equipment is in situ. If you decide to have a funeral service at another venue or location, your family and friends might have to provide the equipment themselves. But I've done several ceremonies in village halls and function rooms where a lap top and screen link up has worked wonders!

As far as photographs are concerned, there is an opportunity to have images of you, your life and loved ones on the Orders of Service (little booklets showing the content of the ceremony), should you or they wish to have them. Funeral directors can get these designed and printed (for a fee) or some families produce their own, more personal versions. You can also have photographs on display at the ceremony venue, as well as at the refreshments afterwards. And there is an option for an on-screen slide show which could also incorporate video footage of you – perhaps at your wedding, on holiday, a sporting event or family get-together. I recently saw a visual tribute which ended with footage of a woman waving from a train while on holiday in the Alps in the 1970's. It was incredibly moving…

You may not want images of yourself popping up all over the place on the day. Alternatively, you may have some favourite photographs which show you at your happiest (you chose some of these in Part One) and you might want to make a note of them and let your loved ones known where they are. You may want to go as far as recording a message for everyone to hear on the day. This could be just a voice recording or a video of you (we'll talk more about messages a little later).

A Gentle Word Of Caution…

All these new choices are a wonderful thing and add a whole new level of meaning and memories on the day. But they can, of course, be highly emotive. I am often moved to tears by visual tributes – and that's coming from someone who is not related to the person in any way. I tend to position myself so that I can't be seen and make sure I pull myself together before I'm 'back on' as it were. It does help enormously if there is a happy song playing alongside rather than anything too mournful or heartbreaking.

So my advice on this would be, if any of the above appeals to you, express your wishes but perhaps add a note for your loved ones acknowledging that they may want to decide how much they see of you on the day itself and how much they may wish to view privately as a family or in a gathering of close friends at another time. I'm not telling you what to do – this is, after all, all about YOU and YOUR wishes – I'm just sharing my experience. A life celebration filled with photos and film can be indescribably fantastic, it just needs a little bit of extra consideration – depending on circumstances – when the time comes.

"All photographs are memento mori. To take a photograph is to participate in another person's mortality, vulnerability, mutability. Precisely by slicing out this moment and freezing it, all photographs testify to time's relentless melt."

Susan Sontag

SECTION FIVE
Meaningful Words

Your Life Story

"Let us endeavour so to live that when we come to die even the undertaker will be sorry."
Mark Twain

This is, perhaps, the most important aspect of any funeral ceremony – sharing someone's life story in a meaningful, relevant, accurate way. It's certainly the part I spend most time on in terms of questions I ask when visiting a family, when I'm writing the ceremony, and delivering the ceremony on the day. Because how can we remember a life, celebrate a life, say farewell to a life, without first reminding everyone what that life meant – to the person themselves and to their loved ones?

We all mean different things to different people. Family and friends will share their feelings about their loved one with me when I meet them. They may also decide to share those feelings and memories with everyone else, in person, on the day of the funeral, rather than ask me to speak on their behalf. And it's wonderful to have that perspective. They can take comfort, and pride, in being able to pay tribute to you, while everyone else can call to mind their own memories and, hopefully, learn something new about you too. BUT what would be equally – perhaps even more – meaningful would be to know what your life meant to you. What were your most significant events, achievements and experiences? Who mattered to you? How would you like to be remembered? And, of course, you already have all this information at your fingertips because we covered so much of this in Part One.

I've listed again some of the main headings and questions we covered earlier, to help you. Remember it would be nice if you could share these memories with your loved ones in person. People regularly tell me “I wish I’d asked Dad about his school days” or “I’d love mum to have told me how she met my dad”.

And if, during this process, you recalled old friends, colleagues, neighbours, who you are still in touch with, remember to make sure your family have contact details so they can be notified when the time comes and have the opportunity to come and say farewell to you on the day.

Early Life

- Where and when were you were born?
- What were you parents’ names?
- Where did you grow up?
- Do you have brothers and sisters?
- Any specific early childhood memories?

Education

- Where did you go to school?
- What did you enjoy and what did you dislike?
- Can you name any friends?
- Did you go on to further education?
- Any particular qualifications?
- Were there any formative experiences?
- Any influences on your career choice?

Relationships

- Has there been a significant other, or others, in your life?
- How and where did you meet?
- Did you marry? If so, where and when?
- Do you have children? Are you a grandparent?
- Any other important relationships in your life – parents, siblings, cousins, nieces, nephews?
- Are there friendships which have meant a great deal?
- Memorable pets?

Working Life

- What have you spent your working life doing?
- Any particular employers or organisations?
- What have you enjoyed most?
- Any jobs you really disliked?
- Any memorable bosses or colleagues?
- Any work memories you'd like to share?
- Proud moments?

Interests

- Do you have any particular interests, hobbies, talents?
- Have you enjoyed music, gardening, sport, cinema, reading, crafts, TV shows, socialising, theatre, fitness, cooking,walking…
- Any clubs, groups, volunteer organisations you've belonged to?

Travel

- Where in the UK/World have you lived and worked?
- Where have you travelled to?
- Any memorable holidays or overseas experiences?

Proudest moments

- What or who have you been most proud of in your life?

How would you describe yourself?

- If you had to describe yourself in five words – capturing your character and qualities – what would you say?
- What have your values been in life?
- What has mattered most to you?

How would you like to be remembered?

- Is there something in particular you'd like to be remembered for?
- Any links people may make with you?
- Any sayings you've been known for?

Poems and Readings

"The *poetry of the earth is never dead."*
John Keats

Sometimes, the feelings you have or the things you want to say can be found, encapsulated beautifully, in the words of a poem, reading or piece of prose. If you have seen something that reflects these sentiments, or you have a favourite poem or piece of writing that you have always loved, then write down the name of the piece and its author and keep a copy with your notes. You may like to have it read at your ceremony or perhaps hear a lovely audio version – plenty of classic poems and novels have been recorded by the likes of Judi Dench or Alan Rickman. A favourite piece of prose read by a favourite performer would certainly be a nice touch.

A Personal Message

People often ask me what is the most moving or meaningful aspect of being involved in a funeral ceremony. And I think, alongside the privilege of helping people say farewell to their family and friends, is the opportunity to speak also on behalf of their loved one. During my time as a funeral Celebrant I've shared messages – sometimes from people I've met who have been terminally ill, or people I haven't met but who have asked for their words to be shared on the day. This is always very powerful and emotive – first of all for the people gathered together who may not have expected such a message, and secondly for me because I need to do justice to those words while keeping my own feelings in check. But I can say, hand on heart, it has always been a very special moment for everyone involved.

Do you have a message of love, comfort, hope, or gratitude you'd like to share with your family and friends? Perhaps telling them what they have meant to you, and what your hopes are for their lives to come? It's not an easy thing to write… where on earth do you begin? But even a sentence or two may make all the difference to how people feel on the day, and how they learn to live without you. Perhaps you could share a few of those words of wisdom, which we discussed in Part One.

SECTION SIX

Final Thoughts

Donations

"The level of our success is limited only by our imagination and no act of kindness, however small, is ever wasted."

Aesop

Would you like to live on through the good work of others? Is there a charity you support? Or an organisation that means something to you? Most funerals these days provide an opportunity for people to donate to charity. Sometimes those charities reflect the manner in which a person died (Cancer Research UK), or help they received (The Air Ambulance). Contributions may also go towards the places in which loved ones were cared for (Hospice Funds). Or sometimes donations reflect the interests of the person themselves (English Heritage) or causes they care about (NSPCC). If you have a charity you feel reflects you or your interests in some way, you might want to make a note of it. It's not unusual for donations to be divided between two organisations, so there could be one of your choosing and one more fitting, chosen by your family, when the time comes.

Something To Remember You By

"Cover me with soft earth and let each handful be mixed with seeds of jasmine and lilies. And when they grow above, they will breathe the fragrance of my heart into space, and reveal even to the sun the secret of my peace."

Khalil Gibran

Several years ago I did a funeral ceremony for a 60-year-old woman who'd had cancer. She wanted to be remembered in a positive way, not associated with illness, but happy and healthy.

She loved her garden and flowers, so she asked for lilly bulbs to be handed out to people at the end of her ceremony, so they could plant these bulbs and think of her each time they bloomed. A beautiful gesture and much appreciated by everyone, including me. I too was given a bulb and every year a gorgeous lilly unfurls its petals and I think of that lovely lady and her family.

There have been similar gestures requested by individuals or their families over the years… from packets of forget-me-not seeds, to tea bags and golf balls. One lady who was terminally ill even knitted dozens of little sunflower heads which her family turned into brooches for everyone. There is no pressure to do any of this, of course. It's just another idea which may appeal to you. Just remember how you felt about some of those mementos and hidden treasures you've held on to over the years – reminders of the special people in your life. Sometimes the smallest things can make a big difference.

Raising A Glass

"I walk down memory lane because I love running in to you."

Gathering together to share food and drink in the company of loved ones and friends is a vital element as we mark the key stages and events of life – from birthdays, anniversaries and Christmas, to weddings, new arrivals, and, inevitably, departures. Refreshments after a funeral ceremony give family and friends an opportunity to relax together, comfort each other, catch up on missing years, raise a glass in your honour, and, of course, continue sharing memories of you, without the restrictions of ceremony timings or wondering what may be 'appropriate' in a funeral setting.

Refreshments can take the form of anything from a cup of tea back at the family home to buffets at local venues, such as pubs or hotels, or even a picnic on the beach. Where you gather may depend on the type of funeral you've had – you may have a ceremony and refreshments in the same venue or travel from one to another. Ideally this doesn't want to be too far away or complicated for people to find who aren't familiar with the area. Cost will also play a part. Some families can afford waiter service at the golf club, while others enlist the help of friends to bake cakes and make a few sarnies. Either way, it's the gathering of people that matters. You may have a favourite watering hole where you'd like everyone to gather after your ceremony. Perhaps you have a favourite cake that everyone can enjoy a slice of or a much-loved tipple that can be shared out, whether that's a Mint Bailey's or a hot brew.

A Gentle Reminder…

Such is the unpredictability of life, we don't really know who will be there to carry out our wishes but, whoever it is, they will certainly be faced with the considerations of cost (even if you've set some money aside for your funeral). They will also have to consider dates and timings for the ceremony, and, assuming they are your loved ones, be able to make their own mark on proceedings – to have their feelings and tributes expressed in some form on the day.

So, if you are planning a four-hour extravaganza with dancing horses and fireworks but want a crematorium ceremony, you may have a problem. The same goes for a sit-down meal and champagne for everyone on a budget of £2 per head. And if you have chosen everything down to the very last flower and written all the words, can anyone else have an input? I am exaggerating (possibly!) and I'm sure you don't need me to tell you not to bankrupt your precious family or break any hearts. Just a gentle reminder in case that £30,000 marble coffin with your hand-carved image on the lid had made it on to your wish list…

Sharing Your Wishes

While you've been brave enough to look to the future, not everyone is going to be ready to discuss your choice of coffin or final resting place, especially the people who love you and want to keep you in their lives for as long as possible. So here are a few suggestions for how to make your wishes known to the people who matter…

- If they know you've been reading this book then that's an easy way to get the conversation going.

- If the news that you've been thinking about your funeral ceremony comes out of the blue, it might be wise to pick your moment to open up the discussion. Perhaps if a celebrity has passed away, or a story-line in a TV soap or drama covers end of life matters or a funeral ceremony, you could say "That's what I'd like…" or "I'd want my flowers to be white not red" or whatever… You might find yourself on a car journey and pass a sign for a natural burial ground or hear one of your music choices on the radio. Just pass comment and see if you can get a conversation going.

- If you think they can be told you've given it some thought, but going into detail will be too much, then simply tell your loved ones that you've written some of your wishes down, that they are being kept in X place, and you're happy to go through them at any time. Do your best, of course, to reassure them that all is well and you're just being organised.

- This might not be a conversation you wish to have now, and that's fine. Just make sure your wishes can be found when the time comes.

It goes without saying that your wishes should be observed – both morally and legally – provided, as we've said all along, they follow the relevant guidelines. So if you have any concerns you can, of course, lodge your wishes with the executors you have nominated to carry out the instructions of your Will.

And Finally…

Well done you! I think it's fitting that you take a moment to congratulate yourself. Not everyone has the courage to face the inevitable and no matter how much or how little you've planned or written down, you have acknowledged – perhaps even embraced – the prospect of your own funeral. That's a wonderful thing.

I'm hoping this experience has given you peace of mind knowing your farewell wishes accurately and meaningfully reflect the person you are and how you'd like to be remembered. And, I hope, you are left with an overwhelming surge of gratitude for the years you've lived and the life still to come. Now you can put those wishes to one side and focus on the present, doing the things you love with the people you love. That's what really matters…

Remember Me set out to show how we are all extraordinary in our own way. But sometimes we're too busy lurching from one day to the next to realise it. So, whoever you are, wherever you've been, wherever you're going next, and however you want to be remembered, don't ever forget how much you matter. Because it just won't be the same here without you…

"What will survive of us is love."
Philip Larkin

CONCLUSION: WHERE NOW?

"Happiness is not a goal. It's a by-product of a life well lived."
Eleanor Roosevelt

We all want to be happy don't we? It's the feeling we aim for, the state we hope to achieve, the sometimes elusive, utopian place we head off in search for. But I think that search for happiness - the quest for the meaning of life - is a bit like someone turning the house upside down to find their glasses, when the glasses are sat on their head. Because we already have the answer - it's our mortality that gives life meaning. We spend so much time looking for meaning in all the wrong places and worrying about the things we don't know. When what we do know - for absolute certainty - is that one day we won't be here anymore. And the sooner we come to terms with that fact, the sooner we can all know what it means to truly live, and leave behind a positive trace.

As I said at the start of this book, if we can overcome the fear of acknowledging our mortality, we can really make the most of the years we have, appreciate our unique place in the world and create a meaningful legacy that will keep our memory alive in the years to come. And if you embrace your life, celebrate who you are, appreciate how far you have come and approach the future with enthusiasm, curiosity and gratitude, then happiness will not only follow you on your journey of life, it will carry your bags, shine a light on the path and always find you a room with a view.

I can testify to the positive impact mortality awareness brings. I deal with death, bereavement and funerals every day of the working week. And these constant reminders of the fragility of life, how irreplaceable we all are and how much we mean to each other, have given me a whole new perspective on what really matters. I'm a happier person because of it. And I hope that reading this book, taking part in the process of thinking about your life and how you want to be remembered, has a positive effect on you too.

"Begin doing what you want to do now. We are not living in eternity. We have only this moment, sparkling like a star in our hand and melting like a snowflake."

Francis Bacon

ABOUT THE AUTHOR

As a Funeral Celebrant, Nicola Dela-Croix has created and led over 1,000 life celebration ceremonies, gaining a wealth of experience in the funeral and bereavement sector. Now she is using her skills and experience to show people how to create their own unique life celebrations and raising awareness of the positive benefits of engaging with our mortality. Before becoming a Celebrant, Nicola also enjoyed a successful 15 year career as a magazine journalist and editor for some of the UK's best-selling special interest publications. She lives in the village of Helpston in Cambridgeshire with her partner Ped.

Printed in Great Britain
by Amazon

74322466R00061